Keto in 30 Minutes

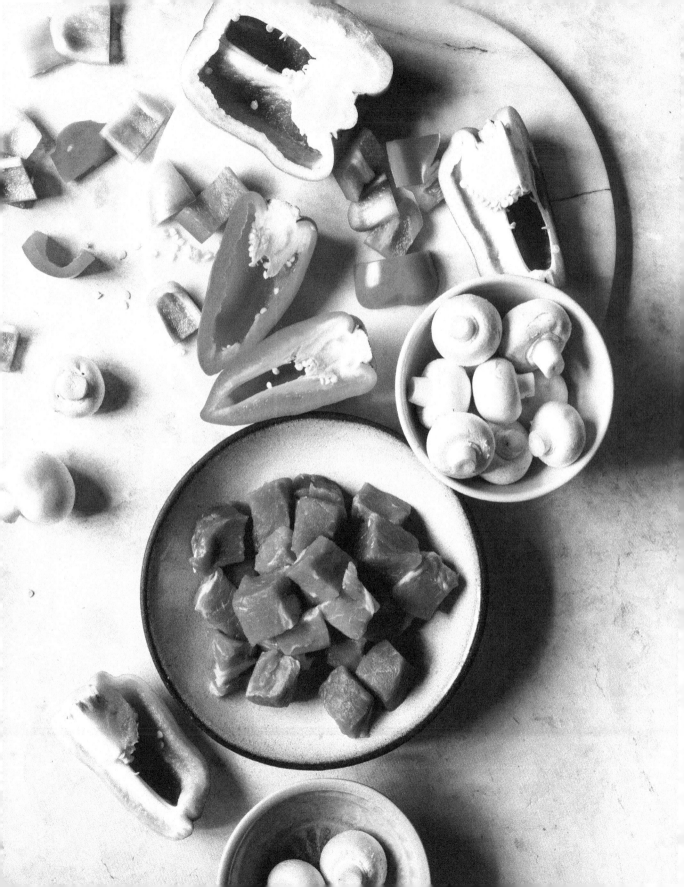

Keto

in 30 Minutes

100 NO-STRESS KETOGENIC DIET RECIPES TO KEEP YOU ON TRACK

EDITED BY **JEN FISCH**

ROCKRIDGE
PRESS

For general information on our other products and services or to obtain technical support, please contact our Customer Care Department within the United States at (866) 744-2665, or outside the United States at (510) 253-0500.

Rockridge Press publishes its books in a variety of electronic and print formats. Some content that appears in print may not be available in electronic books, and vice versa.

Cover photography © 2018 Marija Vidal, food styling by Cregg Green. Interior photography pp. ii, vi, viii, 10, 40, 78, 102, 116, 130, 144 © 2018 Nadine Greeff; pp. 22, 24 © 2018 Hélène Dujardin, food styling by Tami Hardeman; p. 60 © 2017 Linda Schneider. Author Photo © 2018 Suzanne Strong.

Cover Recipes: Sesame Pork & Green Beans, p. 92 with Cauliflower Rice, p. 118

ISBN: Print 978-1-64152-462-9 | eBook 978-1-64152-461-2

CONTENTS

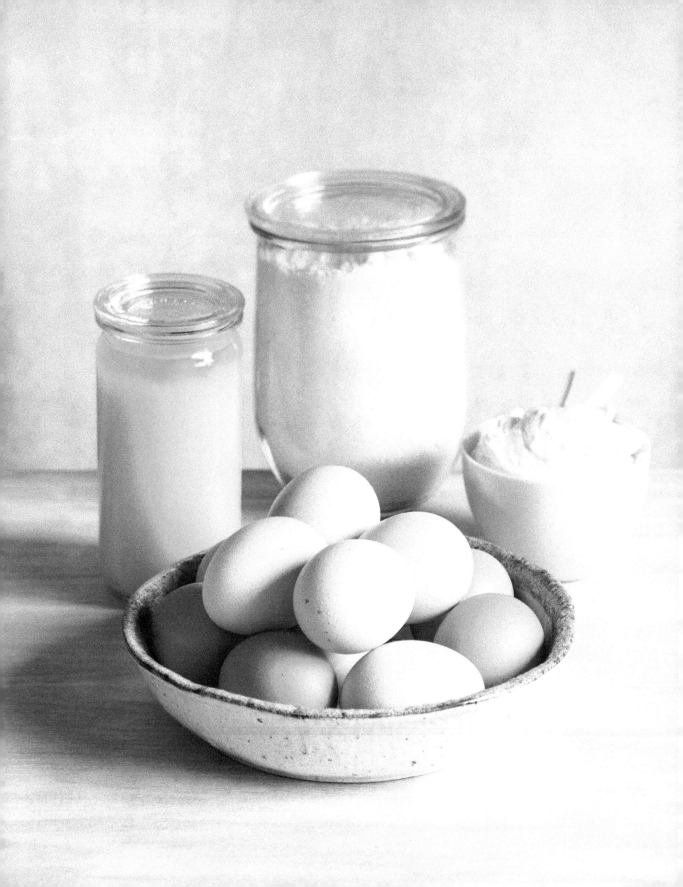

INTRODUCTION

I LOVE TO COOK, but as a single working mom I like to be able to get a delicious keto-friendly meals on the table FAST. I don't have time for super-long or complicated recipes and I'm guessing you don't either! That's why I was so excited to get the chance to pull together a great collection of 100 simple and delicious recipes for *Keto in 30 Minutes.* These recipes show you how practical and sustainable a keto lifestyle can be, even for the busiest people.

I found the keto lifestyle a little over 3 years ago. I was looking for a solution to reduce inflammation in my body caused by two autoimmune disorders, and I was also looking to lose weight. Within a couple weeks I felt a noticeable difference in my systematic inflammation and also on the scale. I became officially hooked on keto and have never looked back. I've lost 40 pounds along my journey. Now I use food for healing.

If you're like a lot of people just beginning keto, you might feel intimidated by cooking and eating in such a different way than you are used to, but you don't need to be. Over the last 3 years I have tested and created hundreds of keto recipes. My main requirements are that they are quick, easy and kid-approved. All of the recipes in this book pass that test!

This book has 7 chapters of recipes to cover every meal in the day, along with all of the info you need to become a ketosis expert. There are a lot of new terms when you are new to keto—macros, ketosis, net carbs, keto flu, and more—so the Keto in a Nutshell chapter will help explain it all. Additionally, you will find lists of foods to enjoy and avoid along with a pantry prep section that will help make shopping and meal prepping simple. There is also a handy chart that shows low-carb alternatives for some of your favorite high-carb foods. Like I said, all the info you need!

There is nothing better than food that tastes good while also helping you reach your health and wellness goals. I'm excited to see which recipes from *Keto in 30 Minutes* become your personal favorites.

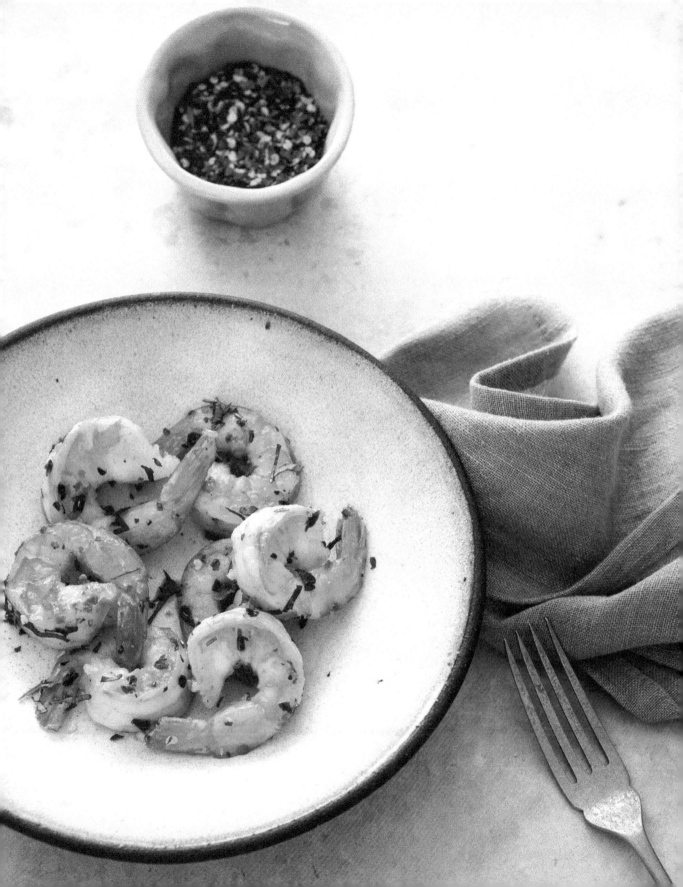

PART I
Ketogenic Diet 101

Shrimp Scampi, page 87

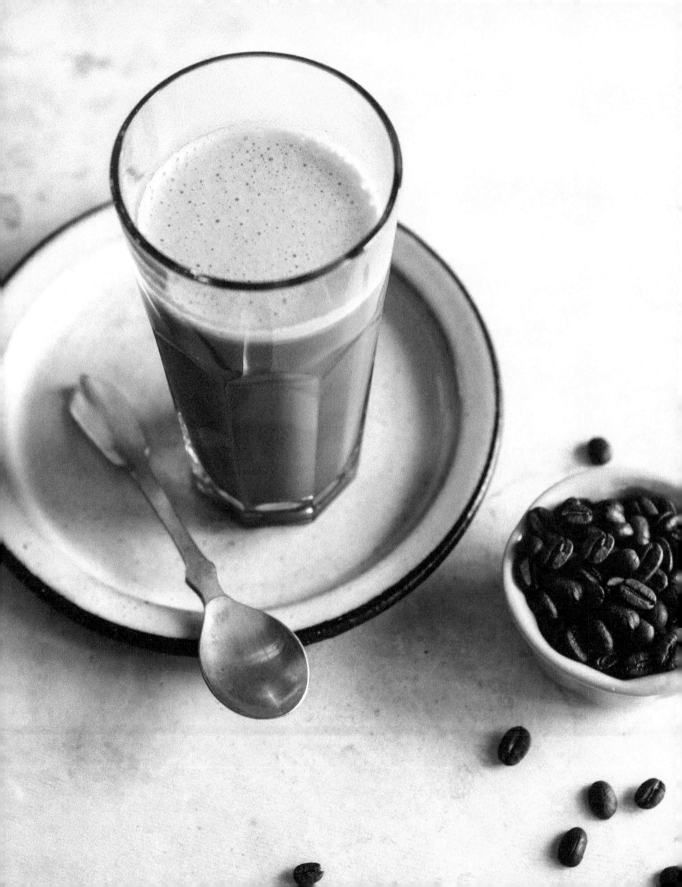

1

Keto in a Nutshell

Bulletproof Coffee, page 42

At its core, the ketogenic diet is all about making your body burn fat—instead of carbs and protein—for fuel. Sound complicated? Actually, it's pretty simple: focus on eating lots of healthy fats and moderate amounts of protein, and keep your carbohydrate intake low (or cut carbs out altogether).

In this chapter, you'll learn the basic science behind this diet, easy-to-follow guidelines to help keep you on track, and the myriad benefits you will experience once you adapt to the keto lifestyle. You'll also find a handy list of keto-approved foods (and those to avoid). Once you understand the principles of the diet, you will be amazed at how easy it is to stay on track, both at home and while you're out and about!

What Is the Ketogenic Diet?

The ketogenic diet can be as simple or as complicated as you make it. In its simplest form, it can be described as staying in ketosis. Ketosis is the process by which your body creates ketones for energy in the absence of carbohydrates. Cave people didn't indulge in boxes of mini brownies; they got their energy from vegetables, berries, and meat. To get in and stay in ketosis, most ketoers start by eating fewer than 20 net carbohydrates per day. Ketogenic dieters also try to keep their daily macronutrient intake (or "macros") at about 5 percent carbs, 20 percent protein, and 75 percent fats. You'll see this is easier than you think. Once you determine how many carbs you can consume before kicking yourself out of ketosis, you may find you can raise the bar from 20 to 50 net carbohydrates per day.

Back when men and women foraged for food, they hunted birds and animals, caught fish, and snagged fruits and berries off plants. With the discovery and refinement of sugar, energy could suddenly be produced from carbohydrates, which are easy to process and turn into energy.

However, they also burn off—and are thus wasted—just as quickly. Before humans began ingesting refined sugar and carbohydrates, we were always in ketosis. Paleo advocates suggest that back then, our bodies were fueled by ketones for energy and burned fat for fuel. Even today, significant amounts of carbohydrates aren't needed. In fact, according to a 2002 study published in the *Journal of Pediatrics*, babies are born in ketosis and stay that way for as long as they're breastfeeding. This also happens to be the time when babies' brains are growing at a tremendous rate. You may not feel hungry while in ketosis because your food is digested and energy is burned more slowly. Basically, you're getting more bang for your food buck.

The ketogenic diet was not developed for weight loss but as a very real remedy for patients with epilepsy, and it is recommended by the Epilepsy Foundation. But, according to a 2004 study published in the *Journal of the International Society of Sports Nutrition*, a ketogenic diet does support weight loss. Indeed, many weight-loss diets were built upon its principles. Paleo can be considered ketogenic, but anyone consuming honey and quinoa is not likely in ketosis either. In some ways you could call the ketogenic diet the blueprint for all low-carb diets. People have used it successfully for weight loss, but also for reducing anxiety and increasing energy and mental clarity. In addition, a 2013 study published in the *European Journal of Clinical Nutrition* showed that it may even help prevent acne, Parkinson's disease, multiple sclerosis, and cancer. No matter your journey, the recipes in this book are ketogenic compliant—meaning they are naturally low in carbs—and may help with one, or all, of the preceding ailments. And your belly will feel full all the while!

GETTING INTO KETOSIS

When eating a high-carb diet, your body is in a metabolic state of glycolysis, which simply means that most of the energy your body uses comes from blood glucose. In this state, after each meal, your blood glucose is spiked causing higher levels of insulin, which promotes storage of body fat, and blocking the release of fat from your adipose (fat storage) tissues.

In contrast, a low-carb, high-fat diet puts your body into a metabolic state called ketosis. Your body breaks down fat into ketone bodies (ketones) for fuel as its primary source of energy. In ketosis, your body readily burns fat for energy, and fat reserves are constantly released and consumed. It's a normal state—whenever you're low on carbs for a few days, your body will do this naturally.

Most cells in your body use ketones and glucose for fuel. For cells that can only take glucose, like parts of the brain, the glycerol derived from dietary fats is made into glucose by the liver through gluconeogenesis. The main goal of the keto diet is to keep you in nutritional ketosis all the time.

For those just starting the keto diet, to be fully keto-adapted usually takes anywhere from four to eight weeks. Once you become keto-adapted, glycogen (the glucose stored in your muscles and liver) decreases, you carry less water weight, your muscle endurance increases, and your overall energy levels are higher than before. Also, if you kick yourself out of ketosis by eating too many carbs, you return to ketosis much sooner than when you were not keto-adapted. Additionally, once you are keto-adapted, you can generally eat up to 50 grams of carbs per day and still maintain ketosis.

KETO NUTRITION

The ketogenic diet is simple in its implementation (goal: stay in ketosis); however, the path can be different for each person. Everyone begins at 20 net carbohydrates and then, over time, determines how many they can consume without being kicked out of ketosis. It's up to each of us to learn what our personal "kick out" point is and stay below it.

How do you know if you are in ketosis? Simple: keto sticks. Tubes of these thin test strips are available at your local pharmacy. Simply urinate on a stick to find out if you're in or out of ketosis. If the stick turns light pink, you're out of ketosis; any shade of purple means you're in. Note that a darker shade of purple does not indicate "better" ketosis—it matters only if you are in or out, burning fat or not. There aren't tiers or levels you need to reach. However, if you're diabetic, you run the risk of a condition called ketoacidosis on a ketogenic diet. Be sure to talk with your doctor about the diet; he or she will likely recommend using keto sticks and making sure you stay in the light purple range.

To calculate net carbohydrates, take the number of carbohydrates you consume and subtract the number of fiber grams consumed. This is the number you'll use to track your daily total. When food is high in fiber, like coconut, you can eat more of it even if the carbohydrate numbers look a little scary. Some people on the keto diet find that paying attention to macros (or daily percentages of foods that fall into the three main macronutrient categories: carbohydrates, proteins, and fat) is helpful for keeping track of their weight loss, and other people use them for medical reasons. If you don't have any medical reasons to stick to certain percentages, then a good daily starting point for the ketogenic diet is 5 percent carbs, 20 percent proteins, and 75 percent fats. If this doesn't keep you in ketosis, try 5 percent carbs, 15 percent proteins, and 80 percent fats.

Ultimately, it's up to you to find the balance that works best for you. There are hundreds of calculators online that you can use to input your stats, such as weight, height, sex, weight goal, and so on, and the calculator will tell you what is supposed to be the ideal macro for you. The amount of carbs (which should generally come from vegetables) or fats that will create ketosis in the body varies for different people. It is certainly not an exact science. See page 150 for a list of macro calculator apps.

DIET GUIDELINES

Following are some of the best ways to stay in ketosis and get the most out of your ketogenic experience. These tips will help you survive what's known as "keto flu." During your first few days, or up to a week, of ketosis, you may feel a bit tired, sluggish, and dizzy as your body adjusts to producing and burning ketones as energy instead of carbohydrates.

Stick to your macros. The daily 5/20/75 ratio is worth sticking to because it works. Too many carbs and you won't burn fat. Too much protein and it won't burn off if you don't use it. Not enough fat and you won't be full. All these problems add up to less energy. The recommended ratio allows for a whole food approach to ketosis that includes alkalizing green veggies, which break down the acids in meat.

Keep your electrolytes up. Electrolytes are the minerals in our blood that keep us hydrated and keep our nerves and muscles working properly in balance. By producing ketones, you'll be flushing out more electrolytes than usual. This means you should increase your salt intake while following keto because your body won't hang onto sodium like it used to. Most ketoers do this by drinking chicken broth or bouillon daily, especially in the first few weeks of ketosis while the body is adjusting. If you feel achy in the first week on keto while going through carbohydrate withdrawal, bouillon helps. Many ketoers use magnesium supplements as well.

Drink lots of water. Drinking water is one of those things that everyone tells you to do, and you don't take it seriously until you end up with a kidney stone! Drinking two to three liters of water every day will make your body feel clean, full, and hydrated; keep your bowels moving; and help you lose weight faster if that's what you're ketoing for.

Keep track of what you eat. Measuring what you eat turns any diet into a game. Use apps like MyFitnessPal to track your meals and measure your macros at the end of the day. There's also an app called Quip you can use to make shopping lists. It includes check marks that allow you to reuse your shopping list every week.

Eat your calories. Don't try to do a low-calorie ketogenic diet, or you'll end up without any fuel. Fat is your new fuel. Without it, you'll not only be hungry, but you also won't lose weight. Many ketoers eat 1,800 calories or more per day and find that eating less than that actually makes them stop losing weight. But don't overindulge, either. You won't likely lose weight eating 5,000 calories a day. The good news is that you won't be hungry enough to eat that much anyway!

Stock up on healthy fats. Fat has become a dirty word in our society. But there are plenty of good fats out there. Cook everything in ghee, which is lactose- and casein-free clarified butter, high in anti-inflammatory omega-3 fatty acids. For times when you run out of this magical golden buttery oil, keep a backup of coconut oil and olive oil. Avoid processed oils like vegetable, sunflower seed, soybean, and corn—they are high in inflammatory omega-6s, which in turn destroy the healthy omega-3s in your body.

Invest in certified organic, grass-fed, and free-range products. Now that your diet is exchanging highly refined carbohydrates for mostly fats and proteins, you'll want to pay extra-special attention to the quality of those ingredients.

Stick to real food, not low-carb products. If you check the label of most low-carb products, unless they're also paleo products, you'll be shocked at their ingredients, such as unpronounceable chemical additives. You can control what goes into your body by making your own meals and sticking to whole foods.

Going Keto?

Maintaining a low-carb, high-fat diet is beneficial for weight loss. Most importantly, according to an increasing number of studies, it helps reduce risk factors for diabetes, heart diseases, stroke, Alzheimer's, epilepsy, and more. The keto diet promotes fresh whole foods like meat, fish, veggies, and healthy fats and oils, and greatly reduces processed, chemically treated foods. It's a diet that you can sustain long-term and enjoy. What's not to enjoy about a diet that encourages eating bacon and eggs for breakfast!

Studies consistently show that a keto diet helps people lose more weight, improve energy levels throughout the day, and stay satiated longer. The increased satiety and improved energy levels are attributed to most of the calories coming from fat, which is very slow to digest and calorically dense. As a result, keto dieters commonly consume fewer calories because they're satiated longer and don't feel the need to eat as much or as often.

In addition to those benefits, eating a keto diet in the long term has been proven to:

- Result in more weight loss (specifically body fat)
- Reduce blood sugar and insulin resistance (commonly reversing prediabetes and type 2 diabetes)
- Reduce triglyceride levels
- Reduce blood pressure
- Improve levels of HDL (good) and LDL (bad) cholesterol
- Improve brain function

Facing the Keto (or Carb) Flu

After a few days on a low-carb or ketogenic diet, you may find yourself fighting something called the carb flu. Basically, this is your body's way of recalculating your metabolism. All of a sudden, you are not processing the foods your body is used to processing, and you are processing higher quantities of other foods.

Think of your GPS when you turn somewhere unplanned. Instead of taking in the foods that are familiar to your body, you are sending in nutrients that your body has to "think" about and use a lot of energy to process. This is a good thing! This means it's working. But, it also means you may feel a little more tired than usual. You might find yourself a little foggier in the brain than normal. You may get a few headaches or even feel nauseous. Drinking a little fresh ginger and lemon steeped in hot water can help with that. Your body is full of enzymes that are waiting for those carbs you usually eat, but they aren't coming in. Now your body has to create new enzymes that will burn fat for fuel instead of carbs. The transition is called the low-carb or ketosis flu.

Give it a few days—or even a week or two—to sort itself out. In that time, continue eating ketogenically, but if you don't feel like doing hard-core exercise, don't. Take walks instead, ride a bike, or play. Some people find that days two and three can be challenging, and scheduling these days to fall on a weekend (or other day with low activity) can be beneficial.

Remember, especially as you're starting out, to keep replenishing your water: tap, distilled, mineral, or sparkling. Drink bone broth (chicken or beef). Eat fats such as avocados and some butter (hold the bread and potatoes). Try not to overeat protein if you're feeling very sick, as doing so can make it worse before it gets better. Fatty meats and cheeses can help ease the transition and ensure that your body doesn't convert the protein to glucose. If you have high blood pressure or cholesterol, you may want to consult with your doctor first. You are teaching your body how to eat in a whole new way!

Here are the basic foods you can use in your everyday cooking, along with the foods you will want to cross off your grocery list. Whenever possible, buy the highest quality versions of keto-approved foods. Though grass-fed meats, wild-caught salmon, and organic produce may be more expensive than their conventional counterparts, natural, sustainably raised/grown foods are free from unnecessary chemicals and preservatives and much more nutrient-rich. Visit your local farmers' market for the best deals on high-quality produce, meats, and dairy.

Foods to Enjoy: High Fat/Low Carb (Based on Net Carbs)

MEATS & SEAFOOD

Beef (ground beef, steak, etc.)
Chicken
Crab
Crawfish
Duck
Fish
Goose
Lamb
Lobster
Mussels
Octopus
Pork (pork chops, bacon, etc.)
Quail
Sausage (without fillers)
Scallops
Shrimp
Veal
Venison

DAIRY

Blue cheese dressing
Burrata cheese
Cottage cheese
Cream cheese
Eggs
Greek yogurt (full-fat)
Grilling cheese
Halloumi cheese
Heavy (whipping) cream
Homemade whipped cream
Kefalotyri cheese
Mozzarella cheese
Provolone cheese
Queso blanco
Ranch dressing
Ricotta cheese
Unsweetened almond milk
Unsweetened coconut milk

NUTS & SEEDS

Almonds
Brazil nuts
Chia seeds
Flaxseeds
Hazelnuts
Macadamia nuts
Peanuts (in moderation)
Pecans
Pine nuts
Pumpkin seeds
Sacha inchi seeds
Sesame seeds
Walnuts

FRUITS & VEGETABLES

Alfalfa sprouts
Asparagus
Avocados
Bell peppers
Blackberries
Blueberries
Broccoli
Cabbage
Carrots (in moderation)
Cauliflower
Celery
Chicory
Coconut
Cranberries
Cucumbers
Eggplant (in moderation)
Garlic (in moderation)
Green beans
Herbs
Jicama
Lemons
Limes
Mushrooms
Okra
Olives
Onions (in moderation)

Pickles
Pumpkin
Radishes
Raspberries

Salad greens
Scallions
Spaghetti squash (in
    moderation)

Strawberries
Tomatoes (in moderation)
Zucchini

Foods to Avoid: Low Fat/High Carb (Based on Net Carbs)

MEATS & MEAT ALTERNATIVES

Deli meat (some, not all)
Hot dogs (with fillers)
Sausage (with fillers)
Seitan
Tofu

DAIRY

Almond milk (sweetened)
Coconut milk (sweetened)
Milk
Soy milk (regular)
Yogurt (regular)

NUTS & SEEDS

Cashews
Chestnuts
Pistachios

FRUITS & VEGETABLES

Apples
Apricots
Artichokes
Bananas
Beans (all varieties)
Boysenberries
Burdock root
Butternut squash
Cantaloupe
Cherries
Chickpeas
Corn
Currants
Dates
Edamame
Elderberries
Gooseberries
Grapes
Honeydew melon

Huckleberries
Kiwis
Leeks
Mangos
Oranges
Parsnips
Peaches
Peas
Pineapples
Plantains
Plums
Potatoes
Prunes
Raisins
Sweet potatoes
Taro root
Turnips
Water chestnuts
Winter squash
Yams

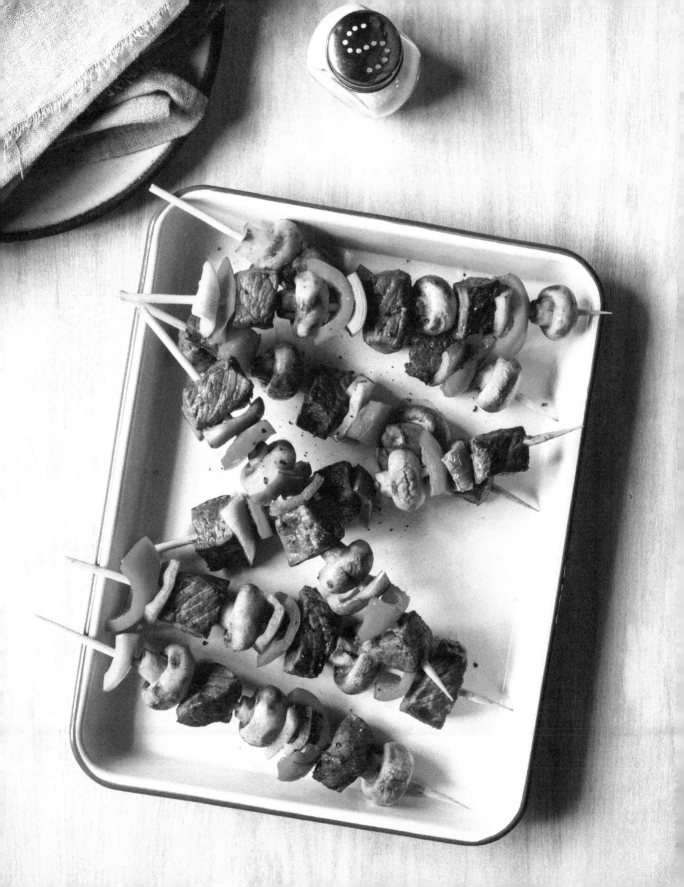

2

Prepping for Success

Tips & Tricks for an Easy Keto Lifestyle

Steak, Mushroom & Pepper Kebabs, page 96

ow that you've brushed up on the science behind the keto diet and learned why it works, it's time to get started and set yourself up for success. In this chapter, you'll learn how to make your kitchen keto-friendly by removing foods that don't fit in the diet and shopping for those that will keep you on track and feeling great.

First, Clean Out Your Pantry

Out with the old, in with the new. Having tempting, unhealthy foods in your home is one of the biggest contributors to failure when starting any diet. To succeed, you need to minimize any triggers to maximize your chances. Unless you have the iron will of Arnold Schwarzenegger, you should not keep addictive foods like bread, desserts, and other non keto friendly snacks around. If you don't live alone, be sure to discuss and warn your housemates, whether they're significant others, family, or roommates. If some items must be kept (if they're simply not yours to throw out), try to agree on a special location to keep them out of sight. This will also help anyone you share your living space with understand that you are serious about starting your diet, and will lead to a better experience for you at home overall (people love to tempt anyone on a diet at first, but it will get old and they'll tire quickly).

Yes, you're "getting rid" of unwanted foods in your pantry, but these foods can feed many others. Please, don't throw them away! Find a local food bank or homeless youth shelter to donate them to.

What about Alcohol?

It's a good idea to avoid alcohol entirely during the 28-day plan. After that, you can work it back into your meal plan. Red wine is a low-carb choice, and there are a number of liquors (unflavored) that have zero carbs. However, drinking alcohol can also cause your metabolism to slow down. Your willpower could suffer, too, and eating more before bedtime may be easier to rationalize. If you're committed to going keto, take at least a week or two to detox your body fully before adding alcohol back in.

Get rid of all cereal, pasta, rice, potatoes, corn, oats, quinoa, flour, bread, bagels, wraps, rolls, and croissants.

Get rid of all refined sugar, fountain drinks, fruit juices, milk, desserts, pastries, milk chocolate, candy bars, etc.

Get rid of beans, peas, and lentils. They are dense with carbs. A 1-cup serving of beans alone contains more than three times the amount of carbs you want to consume in a day.

Get rid of all vegetable oils and most seed oils, including sunflower, safflower, canola, soy bean, grapeseed, and corn oil. Also eliminate trans fats like shortening and margarine—anything that says "hydrogenated" or "partially hydrogenated." Olive oil, extra-virgin olive oil, avocado oil, and coconut oil are the keto-friendly oils you want on hand.

Get rid of fruits that are high in carbs, including bananas, dates, grapes, mangos, and apples. Be sure to get rid of any dried fruits like raisins as well. Dried fruit contains as much sugar as regular fruit but more concentrated, making it easy to eat a lot of sugar in a small serving. For comparison, a cup of raisins has more than 100 grams of carbs while a cup of grapes has only 15 grams of carbs.

Next, Go Shopping

It's time to restock your pantry, refrigerator, and freezer with delicious, keto-friendly foods that will help you lose weight, become healthy, and feel great!

With these basics on hand, you'll always be ready to prepare healthy, delicious, and keto-friendly meals and snacks.

- Water, coffee, and tea
- All spices and herbs
- Sweeteners, including stevia and erythritol
- Lemon or lime juice
- Low-carb condiments like mayonnaise, mustard, pesto, and sriracha
- Broths (chicken, beef, bone)
- Pickled and fermented foods like pickles, kimchi, and sauerkraut
- Nuts and seeds, including macadamia nuts, pecans, almonds, walnuts, hazelnuts, pine nuts, flaxseed, chia seeds, and pumpkin seeds

MEATS

Any type of meat is fine for the keto diet, including chicken, beef, lamb, pork, turkey, game, etc. It's preferable to use grass-fed and/or organic meats if they're available and possible for your budget. You can and should eat the fat on the meat and skin on the chicken. All wild-caught fish and seafood slide into the keto diet nicely. Try to avoid farmed fish. Go crazy with the eggs! Use organic eggs from free-range chickens, if possible.

VEGGIES

You can eat all nonstarchy veggies, including broccoli, asparagus, mushrooms, cucumbers, lettuce, onions, peppers, tomatoes, garlic (in small quantities—each clove contains about 1 gram of carbs), Brussels sprouts, zucchini, eggplant, olives, zucchini, yellow squash, and cauliflower. Avoid all types of potatoes, yams and sweet potatoes, corn, and legumes like beans, lentils, and peas.

FRUITS

You can eat a small amount of berries every day, such as strawberries, raspberries, blackberries, and blueberries. Lemon and lime juices are great for adding flavor to your meals. Avocados are also low in carbs and full of healthy fat. Avoid other fruits, as they're loaded with sugar. A single banana can contain around 25 grams of net carbs.

DAIRY

Eat full-fat dairy like butter, sour cream, heavy (whipping) cream, cheese, cream cheese, and unsweetened yogurt. Although not technically dairy, unsweetened almond and coconut milks are great as well. Avoid milk and skim milk, as well as sweetened yogurt, as it contains a lot of sugar. Avoid any flavored, low-fat, or fat-free dairy products.

The Keto Spice Rack

Herbs and spices aren't just a great way to add zip to your meals; they can also help you in your efforts to lose weight. Different spices and herbs have distinct properties and nutrients. Cinnamon, for example, reduces blood sugar levels and carb cravings. Mustard seed can boost your metabolism, as can cayenne pepper. Turmeric has major antioxidant qualities, and many other herbs and spices can tip the scales in your favor.

- *Anise, ground (for a fantastic licorice flavor)*
- *Basil, dried*
- *Black pepper, freshly ground*
- *Cayenne pepper, ground*
- *Celery seed*
- *Cinnamon, ground*
- *Coriander, ground*
- *Cumin, ground*
- *Dill, dried*

- *Garlic powder*
- *Ginger, ground*
- *Marjoram, ground*
- *Mustard seed*
- *Oregano (the oil of which has amazing healing properties), dried*
- *Salt, preferably sea (iodized)*
- *Thyme, dried*
- *Turmeric, ground*

FATS & OILS

Avocado oil, olive oil, MCT (medium-chain triglycerides) oil, butter, lard, and bacon fat are great for cooking and consuming. Avocado oil has a high smoke point (it does not burn or smoke until it reaches 520°F), which is ideal for searing meats and frying in a wok. Make sure to avoid oils labeled "blend"; they commonly contain small amounts of the healthy oil and large amounts of unhealthy oils.

ABOUT THOSE SWEETENERS . . .

The sweeteners may sound strange if you haven't heard of them before. They both come from natural sources and are safe to use in any quantity.

Stevia is extracted from the leaves of a plant called Stevia rebaudiana. Stevia has zero calories and contains some beneficial micronutrients like magnesium, potassium, and zinc. It's readily available in liquid or powder form online and in most supermarkets. It's much sweeter than sugar, so containers are usually very small—you won't need nearly as much.

Erythritol is a sugar alcohol that is low in calories, about 70 percent as sweet as sugar, and can be found naturally in some fruits and vegetables. Sugar alcohols are indigestible by the human body, so erythritol cannot raise your blood sugar or insulin levels. Several studies have proven it to be safe. Sugar alcohols can sometimes cause temporary digestive discomfort, but out of the few available sugar alcohols like xylitol, maltitol, and sorbitol, erythritol is considered to be the most forgiving and best for everyday use.

Ten Tips for Keeping Keto Costs Down

Paying higher prices for grass-fed, free-range, organic foods buys you peace of mind on the ketogenic diet. These types of products are generally higher in good fatty acids and lower in not-so-great ones. If you're splurging on high-quality products, here's how you can cut costs elsewhere.

1. Buy from a butcher or local farmer. Butcher shops tend to be less expensive than most supermarkets, and you can also get excellent, less-costly cuts like the lesser-known tri-tip. If you're cooking for the whole family or simply want lots of leftovers, make the slow cooker your friend and take advantage of roasts instead of single cuts of meat. If you have ample freezer space, consider buying a whole cow—seriously. Many farmers sell whole, half, or quarter cows and will butcher the meat and vacuum-seal every cut for you.

2. Shop every week. When you come home to an empty fridge, it's hard to resist the urge to dine out or order in. But to do so while following a ketogenic diet usually means you're getting a cheap salad or an expensive steak, and nobody ever goes for the salad when they're hungry after a long day. A well-stocked fridge translates to nutritious meals for far less money than eating out.

3. Create a meal plan. On the ketogenic diet, you won't need most dried and packaged goods. Instead, you'll be buying a lot of fresh produce, meats, and dairy products that don't have a very long shelf life. Plan a week's worth of meals, along with a shopping list, and avoid veering from that list. By following a plan and a list, you'll avoid wasting food by buying only what you need.

4. Shop the sales and cheaper cuts of meat. You don't need to eat grass-fed ribeye steaks every day. If beef isn't on sale, look for less expensive options like chicken legs or pork chops. You can easily feed a family of four for under $5 if you buy meat on sale.

5. Splurge on the essentials now. Buy staples like ghee, coconut oil, pink Himalayan salt (if you can find it), Maldon sea salt, and dried herbs and spices in bulk from discount outlets. Your pantry will be well stocked, and your week-to-week grocery bill won't get blown up with tiny $15 jars of coconut oil at the grocery store. Most of these products have long shelf lives, and a little goes a long way, so it will be a while before you need to restock.

6. Make your own. Lots of recipes call for chicken broth. Next time you roast a chicken, make your own bone broth. Strain the broth through cheesecloth and freeze individual portions for future recipes. Instead of buying fresh herbs every week, make herbal ice cubes. Mince fresh herb(s) and pack them into ice cube trays so that each cube is about ¾ full. Fill the trays with boiling water to blanch the herbs and put them in the freezer. Pop the ice cubes out when they're frozen and store them in freezer bags.

7. Invest in a vacuum sealer. When you buy meat in bulk, make it last longer with a vacuum sealer. I even marinate my meats with spices and herbs (but not salt) before freezing.

8. Focus on cheaper ingredients. A whole food approach to the ketogenic diet doesn't mean meat every night. Tuna salad on romaine lettuce leaves, or slices of tomato and mozzarella drizzled with herbs, olive oil, and balsamic vinegar is far more budget friendly and equally delicious.

9. Buy in season. Imported strawberries are expensive in December, but in the summer you can get them at even the most expensive farm stand for under $3 a container. Buy in season and save on the fruits and vegetables that are abundant at different times of the year.

10. Make recipes with fewer ingredients. I've tried to eliminate unnecessary ingredients, like an herb garnish, unless it serves a culinary purpose other than looking pretty. (Fresh herbs are indeed lovely, but often only a small amount is needed. Freeze the remaining herbs in some water in an ice cube tray, or in a tightly packed and sealed plastic bag.) You can cherry-pick the recipes you make based on the ingredients required. Ingredients that tend to increase the cost of a recipe include fresh herbs, fancy cheeses, and wine.

Time-Saving Tools & Appliances

Preparing delicious recipes is one of the best parts of the keto diet, and it's quite easy if you have the right tools. The following tools will make cooking simpler and faster. Each one is worth investing in, especially for the busy cook.

MUST-HAVE EQUIPMENT

Food scale: When you're trying to hit your caloric and macronutrient goals, a kitchen food scale is a necessary appliance. You can measure any solid or liquid food, and get the perfect amount every time. Used in combination with an app like MyFitnessPal, you'll have all the data you need to hit your goals sooner. Food scales can be found online for $10 to $20.

Food processor: Food processors are critical to your arsenal. They are ideal for blending certain foods or processing foods together into sauces and shakes. Blenders don't cut it, powerwise, for many foods, especially tough vegetables like cauliflower. One great food processor/blender is NutriBullet. The containers you blend in come with lids or drink spouts so you can take them to go or use them as storage. They're also easy to clean, making the whole system extremely convenient. They typically sell for about $80 online.

Spiralizer: Spiralizers make vegetables into noodles or ribbons within seconds. They make cooking a lot faster and easier—noodles have much more surface area and take a fraction of the time to cook. For example, a spiralizer turns a zucchini into zoodles, and with some Alfredo or marinara sauce, you can't tell you aren't eating noodles. Spiralizers cost around $30 and can be found in large retail stores and online.

Electric hand mixer: If you've ever had to beat an egg white by hand until you get stiff peaks, then you know just how difficult it is. Electric hand mixers save your arm muscles and massive amounts of time, especially when mixing heavy ingredients. You can find a decent one online for $10 to $20.

Cast iron pans: They've been used for centuries and were one of the first modern cooking devices. Cast iron skillets don't wear out and are healthier to use (no chemical treatment of any kind), retain heat very well, and can be moved between the stove and oven. They are simple to clean up—just wash them out with a scrub sponge without soap, dry them off, and then rub them with cooking oil. This prevents rust and encourages the buildup of "seasoning," a natural nonstick surface. Many cast iron pans come preseasoned, and this method preserves the coating. You can find them in many retail stores and online for $10 to $80, depending on the brand and size; Lodge is a popular brand, still made in the United States.

Knife sharpening stone: Most of prep time is spent on cutting. You'll see your cutting speed skyrocket with a sharp knife set. It's also a pleasure to use sharp knives. Aim to sharpen your knives every week or so to keep them in good shape (professional chefs sharpen their knives before every use). Sharpening stones cost under $10 and can be ordered online.

NICE-TO-HAVE EQUIPMENT

The kitchen section of any store can be a wonderland. There are so many intriguing gadgets. It's also nice (although not necessary) to have these other tools on hand if you can't resist the lure.

Instant cooking thermometer: Cooking steak and chicken is much easier when you can easily prod the meat and find out whether it's at the level of doneness that you're shooting for. These can usually be found for $10 to $20 in most retail stores or online.

Measuring spoon set: Get the right amount of an ingredient quickly. These sets can go from $5 to $10 in any supermarket, store, or online.

Tongs: Tongs reduce splatter when working quickly (compared to using a fork or spatula to flip something in a hot pan). It's best to get tongs with nylon heads so you don't scratch any of your pots or pans. You can get a pair online or in retail stores for $10 to $15.

Use These Tips for Quick, Stress-Free Meals

A little prep work and planning on Saturday or Sunday can make all the difference mid-week, when the idea of putting dinner on the table makes your head spin. Here are five things you can do in advance to simplify mealtimes throughout the week ahead. (These are also great ways to get your family involved in the keto lifestyle—you'll get it all done quicker if everyone pitches in!)

Plan ahead. Want to get a head start on the week ahead? Sit down and sort out your menu for the week. Once you know what you're going to eat and you have all your ingredients, you can spend around 30 minutes getting it sorted. Depending on how organized you want to be, you can either prep your vegetables and proteins and label them for each day or meal, or you can simply estimate about how many of each prepped vegetable you'll need and put them in zip bags or containers labeled with what's inside.

Cut all of your vegetables ahead of time. Most vegetables can be cut and kept fresh or frozen for the week ahead. Work from your hardest vegetables to cut, like squash or sweet potatoes, and move up to onions (which leave the most odor on the cutting board). Place each item in its own zip bag and label.

Marinate meats. If you know you are eating taco salad or shredded beef or chicken for the beginning of the week, get them marinating now. Place your ingredients, meat, and liquid in a zip bag, and place it flat in the fridge. They'll practically be cooked by Tuesday or Wednesday when you're ready to use them!

Freeze it. If you have more than 30 minutes, make up a dish ahead of time and have it ready for after that Thursday night soccer game. You could easily roast a chicken ahead of time and pull half for chicken salad on Wednesday and eat the other half after you're done prepping for the week on Sunday night. (You must eat some of a chicken you just roasted.)

Don't Forget to Exercise!

Yes, you still have to exercise. But what's really great is that instead of killing yourself just to burn calories, on a keto diet, you're working to build strength and muscle mass instead of worrying about calorie loss.

Walk every day. Walk as much as possible. Park at the back of the parking lot, and walk to the store. Walk around the block on your lunch hour. As a mom, I spend a lot of time waiting for kids to finish their activities. I usually take this time—especially if the rest of my day is extra busy—to go for a walk. I walk 15 minutes out and then 15 minutes back.

Ride a bike. Riding a bike is a fantastic way to strengthen your body and get a cardio workout at the same time. Just holding onto the handlebars, steering, and dealing with bumps works your arms out more than you think—and of course the lower-body benefits are second to none. You don't have to be a serious biker either. Don't worry about getting tight pants and a yellow jersey. The great thing about bikes is you don't even have to go fast to get the benefits!

Lift things. One of the best ways to get lean is to lift things and do some work. You don't have to be a bodybuilder, but doing a kettlebell workout (I use a milk jug filled with water or sand) will give you a great workout—especially in the abs and arms. Lift buckets of water, and carry them out to your garden instead of using the hose. If you have back issues, look into other ways to add resistance to your exercise routine.

Run! Run like someone is chasing you. Then walk for a bit. Then sprint for a bit. A number of studies have shown that doing short bursts of intense exercise is actually better for your weight-loss efforts than long, sustained cardio. So, race to the telephone pole; then walk back. Or race up a hill; then walk down. Doing this for 20 or 30 minutes three or four times a week will bring on the sweat and lower the pounds. Always do what's comfortable for your health. Consult with a doctor if you'd like to add high-intensity running to your routine.

Play! You don't have to do a physical routine to get exercise. Do the dance game on your video game system. Play basketball or soccer. Walk on the beach and look for shells. Play Frisbee with your dog. Just have fun and add movement to your every day. You'll see a difference in how you look and feel.

The Recipes

These recipes were developed strategically to help you set up an effective ketogenic diet, quickly. You'll find breakfasts, lunches, dinners, snacks, and treats to mix and match to meet your macro goals. Each recipe includes variations that allow you to change up flavors, cooking methods, and macros so you'll never be bored and never have to wonder what you're going to make next.

For the sake of time, you won't encounter any hard-to-find ingredients, and all of the recipes come together in about 30 minutes. Adopting a new way of eating can be intimidating, even overwhelming, so this book is here to make it as straightforward, manageable, and enjoyable as possible.

Additionally, every recipe and variation includes nutritional calculations including **total calories, total fat, protein, total carbs, fiber, and net carbs** so you can easily monitor your daily allowances and stay on track. For your convenience, the recipes are also labeled:

- Vegetarian
- Nut Free
- Dairy Free

- Gluten Free
- Paleo
- One Pot / Pan / Bowl

In addition, there are many tips included throughout. So without further ado, let's get started!

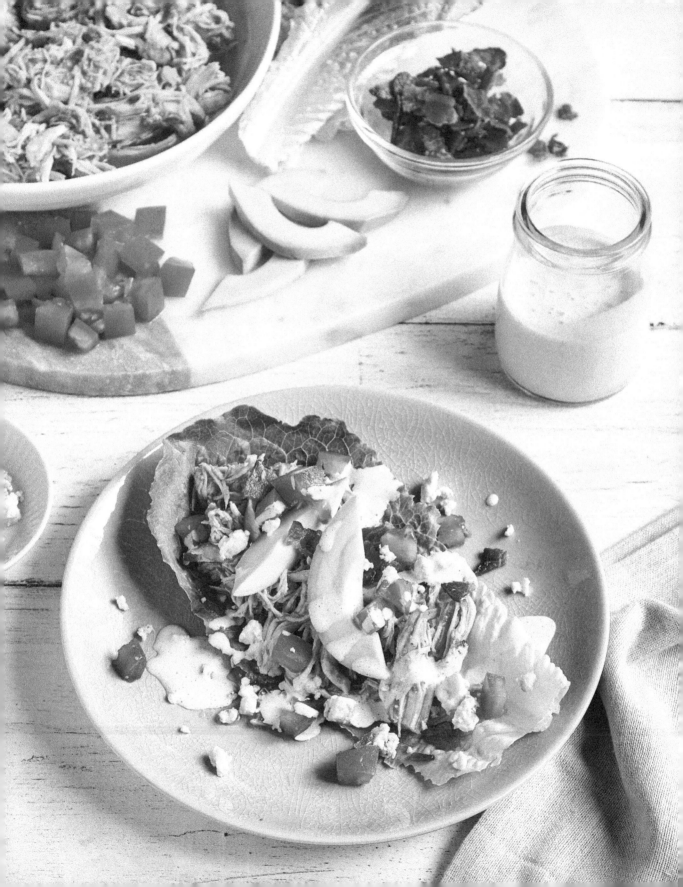

PART II

The Recipes

Chicken Club Lettuce Wrap, page 91

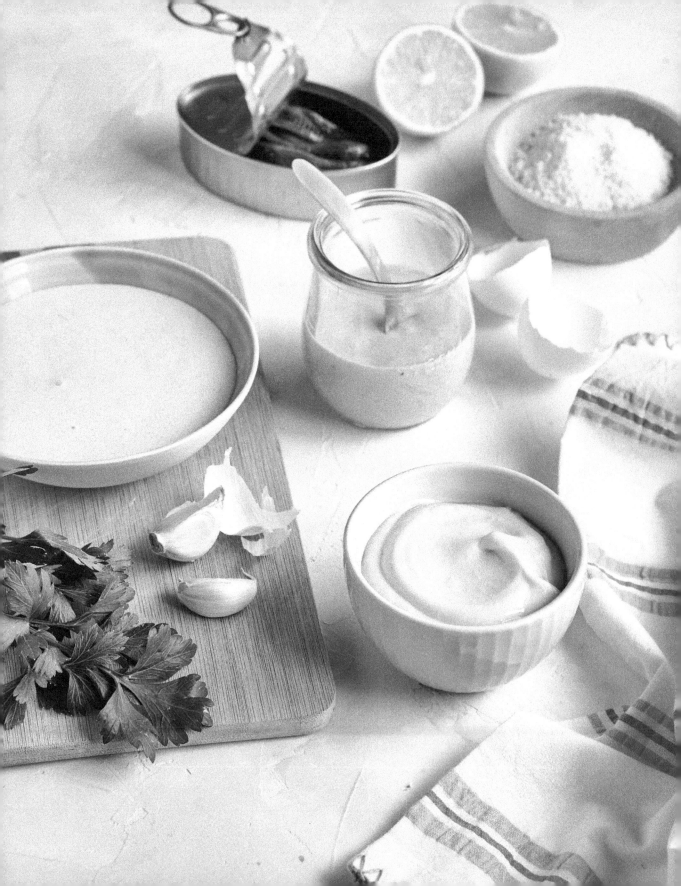

3

Quick Keto Basics

....
Keto Mayonnaise, page 30

Basic Bread

I tried a lot of keto-friendly bread variations until I finally came up with this combination. I love the texture, and it works as a great basic recipe for creating sweet or savory variations.

Serves 12 (makes 1 loaf) | **Prep time: 5 minutes** | **Cook time: 25 minutes**

VEGETARIAN

5 tablespoons unsalted butter, at room temperature, divided

6 large eggs, lightly beaten

1½ cups almond flour

3 teaspoons baking powder

1 scoop MCT oil powder (such as Perfect Keto's MCT oil powder; optional, but it is flavorless and adds high-quality fats)

Pinch pink Himalayan salt

1. Preheat the oven to 390°F. Coat a 9-by-5-inch loaf pan with 1 tablespoon of butter.

2. In a large bowl, use a hand mixer to mix the eggs, almond flour, remaining 4 tablespoons of butter, baking powder, MCT oil powder (if using), and pink Himalayan salt until thoroughly blended. Pour into the prepared pan.

3. Bake for 25 minutes, until a toothpick inserted in the center comes out clean. Slice and serve.

KETO PUMPKIN BREAD VARIATION *Mix all the ingredients together along with ¼ can of pure pumpkin purée. (Make sure you aren't buying sugar-filled pumpkin pie mix; you just want plain pumpkin purée.) Also, mix in 2 to 3 teaspoons of liquid stevia, depending on how sweet you want it, and 1 tablespoon of pumpkin pie spice (a mixture of cinnamon, nutmeg, ginger, and allspice). Bake according to the recipe instructions.*

KETO CHOCOLATE CHIP BREAD VARIATION *Mix the ingredients as instructed, then fold in ½ cup of keto-friendly chocolate chips (such as Lily's).*

Per Slice Calories: 165; Total Fat: 15g, 80%; Saturated Fat: 5g; Protein: 6g, 14%; Total Carbs: 4g, 6%; Fiber: 2g; Net Carbs: 2g; Cholesterol: 106mg

Golden Ghee

Imagine that your cooking oil tastes like butter. That's basically the concept of ghee. Pure, unsalted grass-fed butter is melted to a point where the milk solids, such as casein and lactose, can be removed, leaving a golden oil that can be cooked up to 500°F without burning. Ghee is highly regarded in India, where it is used to cook with but also consumed by the spoonful to aid in digestion. It also has a delightful balance of omega fatty acids.

Makes about 1½ cups | **Prep time: 5 minutes** | **Cook time: 15 minutes**

VEGETARIAN, NUT FREE, GLUTEN FREE, PALEO, ONE PAN

2 cups (4 sticks) unsalted grass-fed butter, such as Kerrygold

1. Cut each butter stick into 10 cubes.

2. In a medium saucepan, heat the butter over medium-low heat until the butter separates and the milk solids fall to the bottom, 10 to 15 minutes. If you want a slightly nutty and rich browned butter flavor, let the milk solids brown just slightly. Otherwise, remove the saucepan from the heat and skim off any foam from the top of the butter.

3. Strain the butter into a jar through several layers of cheese-cloth or a fine-mesh strainer to remove all the solids.

4. Cover the jar and store at room temperature for up to 3 weeks or in the refrigerator for up to 3 months.

Per Serving (1 tablespoon) Calories: 102; Total Fat: 12g; Saturated Fat: 7g, 100%; Protein: 0g, 100%; Total Carbs: 0g; Fiber: 0g; Net Carbs: 0g, 0%; Cholesterol: 30mg

Homemade Nut Butter

Do you know how easy it is to make your own nut butter? All you need is a few minutes, some nuts, and a food processor. To make it even more keto-friendly, this recipe includes some added fat in the form of coconut oil. Use this as a spread for toast, add it to smoothies for added fat and protein, or eat it by the spoonful for a mid-day energy boost.

Makes about 6 servings | **Prep time: 10 minutes** | **Cook time: 0 minutes**

VEGETARIAN, DAIRY FREE, GLUTEN FREE, ONE BOWL

1 cup almonds, pecans, or macadamia nuts
¼ cup coconut oil
Pinch salt (optional)

1. In a food processor, process the nuts for 5 to 10 minutes or until they combine into a butter-like consistency and reach your desired smoothness.

2. Add the coconut oil and process for 1 to 2 minutes more.

3. Add a pinch of salt (if using) and pulse to combine. Serve immediately. Refrigerate leftovers in an airtight container for up to 2 weeks.

CHOCOLATE VARIATION *Add 1 to 2 tablespoons unsweetened cocoa powder when you add the coconut oil.*
VANILLA CINNAMON VARIATION *Add 2 teaspoons vanilla extract and 1 teaspoon ground cinnamon to the nut butter. Stir to combine.*

....

Per Serving (3 tablespoons) Calories: 219; Total Fat: 21g, 83%; Protein: 5g, 8%; Total Carbs: 5g; Fiber: 3g; Net Carbs: 2g, 9%; Sugar: 1g

Chocolate Variation Per Serving Calories: 223; Total Fat: 22g, 82%; Protein: 6g, 9%; Total Carbs: 6g; Fiber: 3g; Net Carbs: 3g, 9%; Sugar: 1g

Vanilla Cinnamon Variation Per Serving Calories: 224; Total Fat: 21g, 81%; Protein: 5g, 9%; Total Carbs: 5g; Fiber: 3g; Net Carbs: 2g, 10%; Sugar: 1g

Whipped Cream

Homemade whipped cream is a million times better than the store-bought variety, and since you're keto, you probably have heavy whipping cream in your refrigerator already. For best results, chill your metal mixing bowl in the freezer for 1 hour before you start the recipe.

Serves 4 │ Prep time: 5 minutes

VEGETARIAN, NUT FREE, GLUTEN FREE, ONE BOWL

½ cup heavy whipping cream

½ teaspoon vanilla extract

1. In a chilled bowl, add the whipping cream and vanilla.

2. Using a hand mixer, mix on low until just combined, then switch to high for 2 minutes, until stiff peaks form.

VARIATION *If you want extra sweetness, add 1 tablespoon of confectioners' erythritol.*

. . . .

Per Serving Calories: 104; Total Fat: 11g, 93%; Protein: 1g, 4%; Total Carbs: 1g, Fiber: 0g; Net Carbs: 1g, 3%

Keto Mayonnaise

This mayonnaise is simple to make, it can be stored for up to a week in the fridge, and it makes for a guilt-free addition to just about any dish. Incorporating mayonnaise into your meal is a great way to stay within your fat goals for the day.

Makes about 2 cups | Prep time: 10 minutes

VEGETARIAN, NUT FREE, DAIRY FREE, GLUTEN FREE, PALEO, ONE BOWL

2 large egg yolks, at room
 temperature
2 tablespoons freshly squeezed
 lemon juice
1 tablespoon apple cider vinegar
1 teaspoon salt
1 teaspoon Dijon mustard
1½ cups olive oil or avocado oil

1. In a food processor, combine the yolks, lemon juice, vinegar, salt, and mustard, and blend for about 30 seconds, or until the mixture thickens.

2. With the food processor on high speed, slowly drizzle in the olive oil in a thin stream until the mixture thickens.

3. Store in a glass jar or airtight container in the refrigerator for up to a week.

SUBSTITUTION TIP *To make this recipe egg free, replace the egg yolks with 2 tablespoons of coconut oil.*

....

Per Serving Calories: 94; Total Fat: 10g; Saturated Fat: 2g, 99%; Protein: 0g, 1%; Total Carbs: 0g; Fiber: 0g; Net Carbs: 0g, 0%; Cholesterol: 12mg

Pico de Gallo

Pico de gallo is a super-easy, super-fresh salsa option. Try it with Cheese Chips (page 111), or add it to eggs or any other dish where you want a pop of flavor. It really goes well with just about anything!

Makes 2 servings | Prep time: 5 minutes

VEGETARIAN, NUT FREE, DAIRY FREE, GLUTEN FREE, PALEO, ONE BOWL

1 small onion, finely diced

2 Roma tomatoes, finely diced

½ jalapeño pepper, finely diced (seeds optional)

½ cup chopped cilantro

1 tablespoon freshly squeezed lime juice

Salt

In a small bowl, toss the onion, tomatoes, jalapeño, cilantro, lime juice, and salt. Serve.

VARIATION *You can add minced garlic to the recipe too, if you wish. Adjust the heat level to taste.*

. . . .

Per Serving Calories: 32; Total Fat: 0g, 2%; Protein: 1g, 13%; Total Carbs: 7g; Fiber: 2g; Net Carbs: 5g, 85%

Herb-Kale Pesto

Nutritional yeast adds a lovely, almost cheesy taste to this pesto, as well as a hearty amount of protein and fiber. Nutritional yeast is also a fabulous source of vitamin B12, which is one of the most prevalent nutritional deficiencies in the world. Vitamin B12 is crucial for many metabolic functions and for help in maintaining both a healthy cardiovascular system and nervous system.

Makes 1½ cups | **Prep time: 15 minutes**

VEGETARIAN, NUT FREE, DAIRY FREE, GLUTEN FREE, ONE BOWL

1 cup chopped kale

1 cup fresh basil leaves

3 garlic cloves

2 teaspoons nutritional yeast

¼ cup extra-virgin olive oil

1. Place the kale, basil, garlic, and yeast in a food processor and pulse until the mixture is finely chopped, about 3 minutes.

2. With the food processor running, drizzle the olive oil into the pesto until a thick paste forms, scraping down the sides of the bowl at least once.

3. Add a little water if the pesto is too thick.

4. Store the pesto in an airtight container in the refrigerator for up to 1 week.

SUBSTITUTION TIP *Try spinach or any other dark leafy green in place of the kale for interesting variations. You can also use any of an assortment of different herbs in the same quantity as the basil in this recipe.*

. . . .

Per Serving (2 tablespoons) Calories: 44; Fat: 4g, 82%; Protein: 1g, 9%; Total Carbs: 1g; Fiber: 0g; Net Carbs: 1g, 9%

Herbed Marinara Sauce

You might have thought rich tomato sauces were off your menu when starting the keto lifestyle, so this recipe might be a nice surprise. There are still tomatoes as the base of the sauce, and the carbs are slightly higher than you might want; however, when combined with other foods such as breaded chicken and mozzarella cheese (as in chicken parm, for instance), the percentages of fat, protein, and carbs are perfect.

Serves 4 | Prep time: 10 minutes

VEGETARIAN, NUT FREE, GLUTEN FREE, ONE BOWL

1 (14-ounce) can unsweetened whole peeled tomatoes

2 tablespoons extra-virgin olive oil

2 tablespoons grated Parmesan cheese

1 tablespoon balsamic vinegar

1 teaspoon chopped fresh basil

1 teaspoon chopped fresh oregano

1 teaspoon chopped fresh parsley

Pinch red pepper flakes

Pinch sea salt

Pinch freshly ground black pepper

1. In a food processor, pulse the tomatoes, olive oil, Parmesan cheese, vinegar, basil, oregano, parsley, red pepper flakes, sea salt, and pepper until the sauce is smooth.

2. Store the sauce in a sealed container in the fridge until you want to use it, and then heat the sauce in a saucepan over low heat.

Per Serving (½ cup) Calories: 96; Fat: 8g, 75%; Protein: 2g, 8%; Total Carbs: 4g; Fiber: 2g; Net Carbs: 2g, 17%; Sugar: 2g

Ranch Dressing

This classic is great as a dip for veggies and breaded meats, and of course as a dressing for green salads. It's really easy to make at home, which helps you cut down on the amount of preservatives you feed your family. If you want, make a big batch of the spice mix so it's ready to go when you need it (it's also a great way to season meat before grilling).

Makes about 1½ cups | **Prep time: 5 minutes** | **Cook time: 5 minutes**

VEGETARIAN, NUT FREE, GLUTEN FREE, ONE BOWL

1 cup Keto Mayonnaise
  (page 30)
½ cup sour cream
1½ teaspoons dried chives
1 teaspoon dry mustard
½ teaspoon dried dill
½ teaspoon celery seed
½ teaspoon onion powder
½ teaspoon garlic powder
Salt
Freshly ground black pepper

Combine the mayonnaise, sour cream, chives, mustard, dill, celery seed, onion powder, and garlic powder. Season with salt and pepper. Stir well to combine and refrigerate in an airtight container with a lid until ready to use. This will keep for about 1 week.

. . . .

Per Serving (2 tablespoons) Calories: 43; Total Fat: 3g, 63%; Protein: 1g, 9%; Total Carbs: 3g; Fiber: 1g; Net Carbs: 2g, 28%; Sugar: 2g

Chunky Blue Cheese Dressing

Nothing's better than this on a wedge salad with bacon, but it's also delicious with chicken wings and fresh cut veggies.

Serves 4 | Prep time: 5 minutes

VEGETARIAN, NUT FREE, GLUTEN FREE, ONE BOWL

½ cup sour cream

½ cup Keto Mayonnaise
  (page 30)

Juice of ½ lemon

½ teaspoon
  Worcestershire sauce

Pink Himalayan salt

Freshly ground black pepper

2 ounces crumbled blue cheese

1. In a medium bowl, whisk the sour cream, mayonnaise, lemon juice, and Worcestershire sauce. Season with pink Himalayan salt and pepper, and whisk again until fully combined.

2. Fold in the crumbled blue cheese until well combined.

3. Keep in an airtight container in the refrigerator for up to 1 week.

INGREDIENT TIP *You can adjust the amount of blue cheese crumbles to use in the dressing. The amount in the recipe makes for a chunky consistency, but feel free to add a little less if you like it smoother.*

. . . .

Per Serving Calories: 306; Total Fat: 32g, 89%; Saturated Fat: 10g; Protein: 7g, 8%; Total Carbs: 3g, 3%; Fiber: 0g; Net Carbs: 3g; Cholesterol 31mg

Herbed Balsamic Dressing

Having a foolproof salad dressing recipe you can whip up on a moment's notice is a cook's essential. Vinaigrettes are not complicated, but you do need the correct ratios to create emulsification between the acid and oil. Balsamic vinegar adds a pleasing sweetness to this dressing, and since a little goes a long way, you won't be getting too many carbs from the vinegar.

Makes 1 cup | **Prep time: 4 minutes**

VEGETARIAN, NUT FREE, DAIRY FREE, GLUTEN FREE, PALEO, ONE BOWL

1 cup extra-virgin olive oil

¼ cup balsamic vinegar

2 tablespoons chopped
   fresh oregano

1 teaspoon chopped fresh basil

1 teaspoon minced garlic

Sea salt

Freshly ground black pepper

1. Whisk the olive oil and vinegar in a small bowl until emulsified, about 3 minutes.

2. Whisk in the oregano, basil, and garlic until well combined, about 1 minute.

3. Season the dressing with salt and pepper.

4. Transfer the dressing to an airtight container, and store it in the refrigerator for up to 1 week. Give the dressing a vigorous shake before using it.

. . . .

Per Serving (1 tablespoon) Calories: 83; Fat: 9g, 100%; Protein: 0g, 0%; Total Carbs: 0g; Fiber: 0g; Net Carbs: 0g, 0%

In-a-Hurry Spice Blends

Having these blends ready to go makes cooking easy and adds flavor to any dish. Use 4-ounce baby food jars to store the different blends, or any airtight container. If you cook a lot, double or triple the blends so you have them on hand. Store them in a cool dry place and shake well before using.

Prep time: 5 minutes

VEGETARIAN, NUT FREE, DAIRY FREE, GLUTEN FREE, PALEO, ONE BOWL

EVERYTHING SEASONING

Makes 5 tablespoons

1 tablespoon sesame seeds

1 tablespoon poppy seeds

1 tablespoon black sesame seeds

2 teaspoons dried minced garlic

2 teaspoons dried minced onion

2 teaspoons sea salt flakes

INDIAN SPICE BLEND

Makes 5 tablespoons

1 tablespoon garam masala

1 tablespoon ground turmeric

2 teaspoons onion powder

2 teaspoons garlic powder

1 teaspoon ground ginger

1 teaspoon ground cumin

1 teaspoon sea salt

½ teaspoon freshly ground
   black pepper

EVERYTHING SEASONING

Combine all the ingredients in an airtight container, shake well, and store at room temperature.

RECIPE TIP *Toast the sesame seeds for a nuttier flavor.*

INDIAN SPICE BLEND

Combine all the ingredients in an airtight container, shake well, and store at room temperature.

. . . .

Everything Seasoning Per Serving (1 tablespoon) Calories: 35; Total Fat: 2.5g, 64%; Saturated Fat: 0g; Protein: 1g, 12%; Total Carbs: 2g, 24%; Fiber: 1g; Net Carbs: 1g; Cholesterol: 0mg

Indian Spice Blend Per Serving (1 tablespoon) Calories: 20; Total Fat: 0g, 0%; Saturated Fat: 0g; Protein: 1g, 20%; Total Carbs: 4g, 80%; Fiber: 1.5g; Net Carbs: 2.5g; Cholesterol: 0mg

Continued

MEDITERRANEAN SPICE BLEND

Makes 5 tablespoons

1 tablespoon dried oregano

1 tablespoon dried rosemary

1 tablespoon dried parsley

2 teaspoons garlic powder

1 teaspoon onion powder

1 teaspoon lemon-pepper
  seasoning

1 teaspoon dried basil

1 teaspoon sea salt

¼ teaspoon red pepper flakes
  (optional)

MEXICAN SPICE BLEND

Makes 5 tablespoons

2 tablespoons chili powder

1 tablespoon ground cumin

2 teaspoons onion powder

2 teaspoons garlic powder

1 teaspoon ground coriander

1 teaspoon paprika

1 teaspoon dried oregano

1 teaspoon sea salt

½ teaspoon freshly ground
  black pepper

⅛ teaspoon cayenne pepper

MEDITERRANEAN SPICE BLEND

Combine all the ingredients in an airtight container, shake well, and store at room temperature.

RECIPE TIP *Muddle or crush the rosemary to break it up into smaller pieces for the blend.*

MEXICAN SPICE BLEND

Combine all the ingredients in an airtight container, shake well, and store at room temperature.

....

Mediterranean Spice Blend Per Serving (1 tablespoon) Calories: 12; Total Fat: 0g, 0%; Saturated Fat: 0g; Protein: 0.5g, 17%; Total Carbs: 2.5g, 83%; Fiber: 1g; Net Carbs: 1.5g; Cholesterol: 0mg

Mexican Spice Blend Per Serving (1 tablespoon) Calories: 29; Total Fat: 1g, 31%; Saturated Fat: 0g; Protein: 1g, 14%; Total Carbs: 4g, 55%; Fiber: 2g; Net Carbs: 2g; Cholesterol: 0mg

Perfectly Cooked Bacon

Who would have thought you could diet and live a healthy lifestyle with bacon involved? I used to keep bacon out of my diet because of the fat content and all the sodium. Remember—uncured, sugar-free bacon is best!

Serves 8 | **Prep time: 5 minutes** | **Cook time: 20 minutes**

NUT FREE, DAIRY FREE, GLUTEN FREE, PALEO, ONE PAN

1 pound sliced uncured bacon

1. Preheat the oven to 400°F. Line a sheet pan with aluminum foil for easy cleanup.

2. Arrange the bacon slices in a single layer on the prepared sheet pan.

3. Bake for 12 to 20 minutes, depending on the thickness of the bacon and how crispy you like it.

4. Transfer the cooked bacon to a paper towel–lined plate to drain.

5. Serve hot with your favorite meal or store in an airtight container in the refrigerator for up to 5 days.

VARIATION *You can also cook bacon on the stovetop. Start with a cold skillet (cast iron preferred) and arrange the bacon slices in a single layer in the bottom. Cook on low for 8 to 12 minutes, or to your desired crispiness.*

Per Serving (2 slices) Calories: 110; Total Fat: 9g; Saturated Fat: 4g, 74%; Protein: 7g, 26%; Total Carbs: 0g; Fiber: 0g; Net Carbs: 0g, 0%; Cholesterol: 20mg

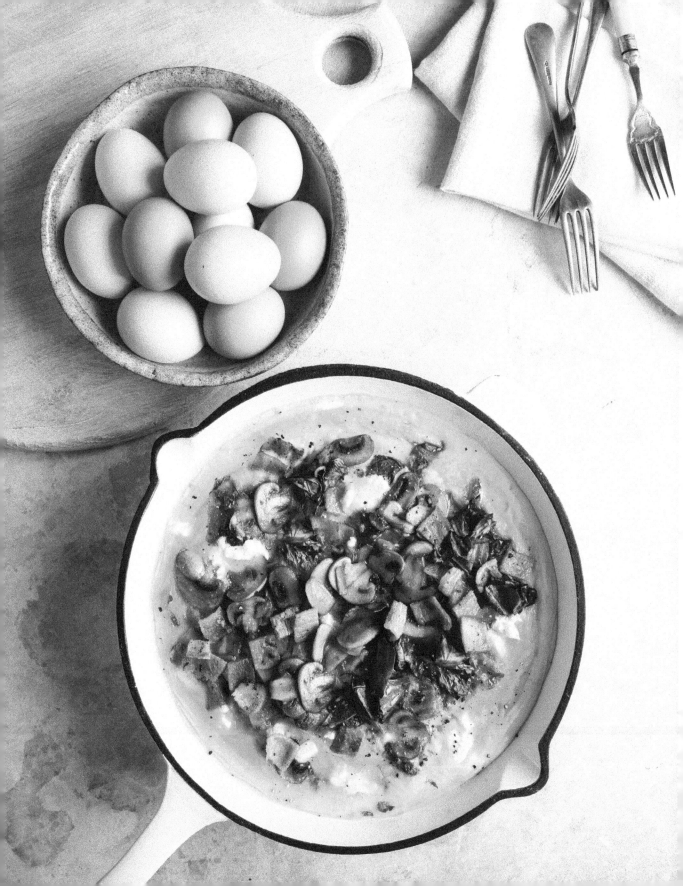

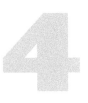

Breakfast

Mushroom Frittata, page 59

Bulletproof Coffee

Bulletproof Coffee is a staple beverage in a lot of keto diets. Though you may be surprised by the ingredient list—butter and oil in coffee?! The added fat plus the caffeine keeps you both full and energized long after you finish your cup.

Makes 1 serving | **Prep time: 5 minutes**

VEGETARIAN, NUT FREE, GLUTEN FREE, ONE BOWL

1½ cups hot coffee

2 tablespoons MCT oil powder or Bulletproof Brain Octane Oil

2 tablespoons butter or ghee

1. Pour the hot coffee into the blender.

2. Add the oil powder and butter, and blend until thoroughly mixed and frothy.

3. Pour into a large mug and enjoy.

RAW EGG VARIATION *To add protein, replace the MCT oil powder with 1 raw egg. It may sound strange, but the egg adds an appealing creamy texture, and although the hot coffee cooks the egg, there will be no hint of cooked proteins.*

PROTEIN AND COLLAGEN POWDER VARIATION *You could also add a scoop or two of protein powder, such as Perfect Keto Collagen, which has a great chocolate flavor that is especially tasty in coffee. The Keto Collagen Powder contains grass-fed collagen, MCT oil powder, and protein powder. The collagen is a good anti-inflammatory addition.*

SPICED VARIATION *Add 1 teaspoon of cinnamon and a little sweetener to your Bulletproof mixture for a delicious spiced version.*

INGREDIENT TIP *If you're new to the keto diet, you will want to start slow with the Brain Octane Oil. It is powerful, so you'll want to work your way up to 2 tablespoons over the course of a few weeks.*

. . . .

Per Serving Calories: 463; Total Fat: 51g, 99%; Saturated Fat: 29g; Protein: 1g, 1%; Total Carbs: 0g, 0%; Net Carbs: 0g; Fiber: 0g; Cholesterol: 61mg

Berry-Avocado Smoothie

This smoothie is delicious and filled with healthy fat, potassium, magnesium, and fiber. Use the liquid stevia if you prefer sweeter smoothies.

Serves 2 | Prep time: 5 minutes

VEGETARIAN, NUT FREE, DAIRY FREE, GLUTEN FREE, ONE BOWL

1 cup unsweetened full-fat coconut milk

1 scoop Perfect Keto Exogenous Ketone Powder in peaches and cream

½ avocado

1 cup fresh spinach

½ cup berries, fresh or frozen (no sugar added if frozen)

½ cup ice cubes

¼ teaspoon liquid stevia (optional)

1. In a blender, combine the coconut milk, protein powder, avocado, spinach, berries, ice, and stevia (if using).

2. Blend until thoroughly mixed and frothy.

3. Pour into two glasses and enjoy.

INGREDIENT TIP *Adding avocado to a smoothie recipe may sound unusual, but it adds nutrition and healthy fat and contributes a creamy smoothness.*

....

Per Serving Calories: 355; Total Fat: 40g; Protein: 4g; Total Carbs: 16g; Net Carbs: 8g; Fiber: 6g

Lemon-Cashew Smoothie

The cashew milk and heavy cream combine to create an absolutely luscious smoothie that is tart enough to be refreshing and still makes for a satisfying breakfast or snack. If you add a few ice cubes, it will be like enjoying a rich citrus sorbet instead of a healthy breakfast. A couple leaves of fresh mint will also enhance the fresh flavor.

Serves 1 | **Prep time: 5 minutes**

VEGETARIAN, GLUTEN FREE, ONE BOWL

1 cup unsweetened cashew milk

¼ cup heavy (whipping) cream

¼ cup freshly squeezed lemon juice

1 scoop plain protein powder

1 tablespoon coconut oil

1 teaspoon sweetener

1. Put the cashew milk, heavy cream, lemon juice, protein powder, coconut oil, and sweetener in a blender and blend until smooth.

2. Pour into a glass and serve immediately.

SUBSTITUTION TIP *Almond milk or coconut milk are also fine choices instead of cashew milk if you prefer those products. Each type of milk adds a slightly different flavor to the smoothie, so try them all to get the right combination for your palate.*

. . . .

Per Serving Calories: 503; Total Fat: 45g, 80%; Protein: 29g, 13%; Total Carbs: 15g; Fiber: 4g; Net Carbs: 11g, 7%

Mean Green Smoothie

Boasting three types of leafy greens, this epic smoothie is perfect for an early morning boost or midday snack. Filled with kale, spinach, and Swiss chard, it provides nutrients like iron, magnesium, calcium, and vitamin C—all of which are necessary for a healthy mind and body. Add herbs like parsley or cilantro for an extra flavor bite.

Serves 2 │ Prep time: 10 minutes

VEGETARIAN, NUT FREE, DAIRY FREE, GLUTEN FREE, PALEO, ONE BOWL

1½ cups crushed ice, divided

1 cup kale, tightly packed, cleaned, stalks removed

½ cup spinach, cleaned, stalks removed

½ cup Swiss chard, cleaned, stalks removed

2 tablespoons coconut oil

2 tablespoons chia seeds

½ cup water

1. In a blender, place ¾ cup of ice. Add the kale, spinach, and Swiss chard. Blend to combine.

2. Add the coconut oil, chia seeds, remaining ¾ cup of ice, and water.

3. Blend for 1 minute, or until smooth, and serve.

TIME-SAVING TIP *Save time on this recipe by using prewashed frozen spinach, kale, and—if available—Swiss chard. If using frozen vegetables, reduce the ice in this recipe by ¼ cup.*

. . . .

Per Serving (½ of finished smoothie recipe) Calories: 293; Total Fat: 23.3g, 71%; Saturated Fat: 12g; Protein: 7.7g, 11%; Total Carbs: 14.6g, 18%; Fiber: 11.2g; Net Carbs: 3.4g ; Cholesterol: 0mg

Cacao Crunch Cereal

Craving cereal without all of the sugar? This healthy combination will give you the crunch and sweetness while also being loaded with fiber and healthy fats. Feel free to add erythritol or a couple of berries for natural sweetness. Strawberries and cacao nibs is a delicious combination!

Makes 2 servings | Prep time: 5 minutes

VEGETARIAN, DAIRY FREE, GLUTEN FREE, PALEO, ONE BOWL

½ cup slivered almonds

2 tablespoons unsweetened shredded or flaked coconut

2 tablespoons chia seeds

2 tablespoons cacao nibs

2 tablespoons sunflower seeds

Unsweetened nondairy milk of choice, for serving

1. In a small bowl, combine the almonds, coconut, chia seeds, cacao nibs, and sunflower seeds. Divide between two bowls.

2. Pour in the nondairy milk and serve.

....

Per Serving (cereal only) Calories: 325; Total Fat: 27, 70%; Protein: 10g, 11%; Total Carbs: 17g; Fiber: 12g; Net Carbs: 5g, 19%

Low-Carb Granola Bars

These on-the-go breakfast bars taste like a treat, but with protein-rich hazelnuts, almonds, and peanut butter, healthy fats, and plenty of antioxidants, they are just the thing to start your morning off right. Make an extra batch to enjoy as snacks throughout the week or on long car rides.

Makes about 12 bars | Prep time: 10 minutes | Cook time: 15 to 20 minutes

VEGETARIAN, DAIRY FREE, GLUTEN FREE

1 cup almonds

1 cup hazelnuts

1 cup unsweetened
   coconut flakes

1 egg

¼ cup coconut oil, melted

¼ cup unsweetened
   peanut butter

½ cup dark chocolate chips

1 tablespoon vanilla extract

1 tablespoon ground cinnamon

Pinch salt

1. Preheat the oven to 350°F.

2. In a food processor, pulse together the almonds and macadamia nuts for 1 to 2 minutes until roughly chopped. (You want them pretty fine but not turning into nut butter.) Transfer them to a large bowl.

3. Stir in the coconut, egg, coconut oil, peanut butter, chocolate chips, vanilla, cinnamon, and salt. Transfer the mixture to an 8- or 9-inch square baking dish and gently press into an even layer. Bake for 15 to 20 minutes or until golden brown. Cool and cut into 12 bars. Refrigerate in an airtight container for up to 2 weeks.

LOW-CARB CHOCOLATE VARIATION *Add 2 tablespoons unsweetened cocoa powder to the bar mix.*

LOW-CARB RASPBERRY VARIATION *If you have room for extra carbs and want to add some fruit, stir in ½ cup chopped fresh raspberries.*

....

Per Serving (1 bar) Calories: 588; Total Fat: 58g, 87%; Protein: 11g, 8%; Total Carbs: 6g; Fiber: 1g; Net Carbs: 5g, 5%; Sugar: 5g

Chocolate Variation Per Serving Calories: 271; Total Fat: 25g, 84%; Protein: 5g, 3%; Total Carbs: 10g; Fiber: 4g; Net Carbs: 6g, 13%; Sugar: 3g

Raspberry Variation Per Serving Calories: 272; Total Fat: 25g, 84%; Protein: 5g, 3%; Total Carbs: 10g; Fiber: 4g; Net Carbs: 6g, 13%; Sugar: 5g

Keto Pancakes

These keto pancakes are a lifesaver when you get a little bored with scrambled eggs (or eggs any style, for that matter). And it couldn't be simpler. You simply throw all the ingredients into a blender then just pour it into the skillet. With just a few ingredients, these pancakes are super simple, super decadent, and totally fit into a ketogenic diet!

Makes 2 servings | **Prep time: 5 minutes** | **Cook time: 10 minutes**

VEGETARIAN

4 eggs

4 ounces cream cheese

¼ cup almond flour

⅔ teaspoon baking powder

⅔ teaspoon ground cinnamon, plus more for sprinkling (optional)

1 teaspoon vanilla extract

1 tablespoon butter, plus more for serving

1. In a blender, combine the eggs, cream cheese, almond flour, baking powder, cinnamon, and vanilla. Blend for about 2 minutes or until all the ingredients are completely combined. Give the blender a shake or tap it on the counter to get rid of any air bubbles in the batter.

2. Heat a large nonstick skillet over medium-high heat. Add some of the butter and stir to coat the bottom and edges of the pan. Pour a small amount of batter into the pan and cook for about 2 minutes until set. (I usually cook two at a time to prevent the pancakes from sticking together or flipping them onto each other.)

3. Flip the pancake(s) and cook for 2 to 3 minutes on the other side. Transfer to a plate.

4. Repeat with the remaining butter and batter. Serve the pancakes immediately with more butter and a sprinkle of cinnamon (if using).

RASPBERRIES AND WHIPPED CREAM VARIATION

Serve this recipe with ¼ cup fresh raspberries (chopped or whole, it's up to you) and some whipped cream—beat heavy whipping cream until thick. Add a few drops (or a packet) of stevia (or other low-carb sweetener) to the whipped cream, if desired.

HAM AND CHEESE CRÊPE VARIATION *Because these pancakes are similar in texture to crêpes, skip the vanilla and cinnamon and serve them with sliced ham and cheese. Roll them up or fold them into triangles and enjoy hot.*

. . . .

Per Serving Calories: 404; Total Fat: 36g, 80%; Protein: 16g, 16%; Total Carbs: 4g; Fiber: 0g; Net Carbs: 4g, 4%; Sugar: 1g

Raspberries & Whipped Cream Variation Per Serving Calories: 470; Total Fat: 42g, 80%; Protein: 17g, 14%; Total Carbs: 6g; Fiber: 1g; Net Carbs: 5g, 6%; Sugar: 2g

Ham & Cheese Variation Per Serving Calories: 492; Total Fat: 40g, 73%; Protein: 28g, 23%; Total Carbs: 5g; Fiber: 1g; Net Carbs: 4g, 4%; Sugar: 1g

Cream Cheese Blueberry Muffins

Blueberry muffins are an ultimate comfort food. Who doesn't remember following the boxed instructions as a kid? Now, you can be transported in a healthier, keto-friendly way with this recipe. And don't forget to slather them with butter before eating!

Makes 6 servings | **Prep time: 10 minutes** | **Cook time: 12 minutes**

VEGETARIAN

Nonstick cooking spray

1 cup almond flour

2 teaspoons ground cinnamon

3 to 4 tablespoons erythritol

¾ tablespoon baking powder

2 large eggs

2 tablespoons cream cheese

2 tablespoons heavy whipping cream

4 tablespoons butter, melted and cooled

2 teaspoons vanilla extract

2 tablespoons blueberries (fresh or frozen)

1. Preheat the oven to 400°F. Spray a muffin tin with cooking spray or line it with muffin liners.

2. In a small bowl, mix the almond flour, cinnamon, erythritol, and baking powder.

3. In a medium bowl, mix the eggs, cream cheese, heavy cream, butter, and vanilla with a hand mixer.

4. Pour the flour mixture into the egg mixture and beat with the hand mixer until thoroughly mixed.

5. Pour the mixture into the prepared muffin cups.

6. Drop the berries on top of the batter in the muffin cups.

7. Bake for 12 minutes, or until golden brown on top, and serve.

SUBSTITUTION TIP *You can replace the cream cheese–heavy whipping cream combination with ½ cup of sour cream.*

Per Serving Calories 160; Total Fat: 15g, 85%; Protein: 4g, 9%; Total Carbs: 10g; Fiber: 2g; Net Carbs: 8g, 6%

Baked Eggs in Avocado

These baked eggs in avocado are a great weekday breakfast you can make quickly before heading out the door. All you do is cut an avocado, scoop some out, and crack in your eggs! Preheat the oven while you're making your morning coffee, and you'll have breakfast before you know it.

Makes 2 servings | **Prep time: 5 minutes** | **Cook time: 15 to 20 minutes**

VEGETARIAN, NUT FREE, DAIRY FREE, GLUTEN FREE, PALEO

1 ripe avocado, halved and pitted

2 eggs

Salt

Freshly ground black pepper

Hot sauce (optional)

1. Preheat the oven to 425°F.

2. Scoop out 1 or 2 tablespoons of avocado flesh from each half and set aside for another recipe. Place the scooped avocado halves in a small baking dish.

3. Carefully crack 1 egg into each half. Season with salt and pepper.

4. Bake for 15 to 20 minutes or until the whites are set and the yolks are cooked to your liking. Sprinkle with some hot sauce (if using) and serve immediately.

GARLIC PARMESAN VARIATION *Follow the recipe as written, but season the eggs in the avocado halves with about 1 teaspoon garlic powder. Top each with 1 tablespoon grated Parmesan cheese and bake according to the instructions.*

SALSA LIME VARIATION *Follow the recipe as written, but top each finished avocado with 1 tablespoon of Pico de Gallo (page 31) and a sprinkling of freshly squeezed lime juice.*

. . . .

Per Serving Calories: 275; Total Fat: 23g, 75%; Protein: 8g, 12%; Total Carbs: 9g; Fiber: 7g; Net Carbs: 2g, 13%; Sugar: 1g

Garlic Parmesan Variation Per Serving Calories: 314; Total Fat: 26g, 74%; Protein: 10g, 13%; Total Carbs: 10g; Fiber: 7g; Net Carbs: 3g, 13%; Sugar: 1g

Salsa Lime Variation Per Serving Calories: 279; Total Fat: 23g, 74%; Protein: 8g, 12%; Total Carbs: 10g; Fiber: 7g; Net Carbs: 3g, 14%; Sugar: 1g

Scrambled Cinnamon & Cream Cheese Eggs

These eggs are a complete keto luxury. You get a pancake-like batch of scrambled eggs topped with some of your favorite sugar-free maple syrup. They're great for dessert, too.

Serves 6 | **Prep time: 10 minutes** | **Cook time: 5 minutes**

VEGETARIAN, NUT FREE, GLUTEN FREE, ONE BOWL

6 tablespoons organic cream cheese, at room temperature

2 tablespoons organic heavy (whipping) cream

3 large free-range eggs

1 teaspoon coconut flour

½ teaspoon ground cinnamon

Sweetener

1 tablespoon Golden Ghee (page 27)

Sugar-free maple syrup

1. In a blender, combine the cream cheese, heavy cream, eggs, coconut flour, cinnamon, and sweetener to taste. Blend until well mixed.

2. In a medium skillet, melt the ghee over medium heat. Pour in the cream cheese and egg mixture. Using a spatula, gently stir the mixture to scramble it until it is cooked through, about 5 minutes.

3. Transfer to a plate and drizzle with your favorite keto-friendly sugar-free maple syrup. Serve immediately.

. . . .

Per Serving (without syrup) Calories: 119; Total Fat: 11g; Saturated Fat: 6g, 83%; Protein: 4g, 13%; Total Carbs: 1g; Fiber: 0g; Net Carbs: 1g, 4%; Cholesterol: 110mg

Egg Breakfast Muffins

These pretty, cheesy muffins are actually quiches baked in a muffin pan without the crust. You can eat them hot out of the oven or chilled, depending on your schedule. These muffins also freeze beautifully, so whip up a double batch for easy meals all month.

Serves 4 | **Prep time: 5 minutes** | **Cook time: 16 minutes**

NUT FREE, GLUTEN FREE

1 tablespoon unsalted butter, for greasing

6 large eggs

1 cup heavy (whipping) cream

½ cup plus 2 tablespoons shredded Cheddar cheese, divided

5 slices cooked bacon, chopped

½ teaspoon chopped fresh cilantro

Pinch salt

Pinch freshly ground black pepper

1. Preheat the oven to 350°F.

2. Lightly grease 8 cups of a muffin pan with the butter; set aside.

3. In a medium bowl, whisk together the eggs, cream, ½ cup of Cheddar, bacon, and cilantro.

4. Season the egg mixture with salt and pepper.

5. Evenly pour the egg mixture into the muffin cups.

6. Bake the muffins until they are cooked through and lightly browned, about 15 minutes.

7. Remove the muffin pan from the oven, and change the oven heat to broil.

8. Sprinkle the remaining 2 tablespoons of Cheddar onto the muffins; broil until the cheese is melted and bubbly, about 1 minute; and serve.

TIME-SAVING TIP *You will be using bacon regularly in a ketogenic lifestyle because it provides a good ratio of fat and protein. Cooked bacon will keep for at least 1 week in the refrigerator, so cook up an entire pack so you can save time when you need to add this product to your recipes in cooked form.*

Per Serving (2 muffins) Calories: 346; Total Fat: 31g, 79%; Protein: 15g, 19%; Total Carbs: 2g; Fiber: 0g; Net Carbs: 2g, 2%; Sugar: 1g

Roasted Asparagus, Bacon & Egg Bake

This is a complete meal with eggs, crispy bacon, and oven-roasted asparagus in just one skillet. If you are short on time and want to skip a step in this recipe, use a sheet pan instead of a skillet. Lay out the prepped asparagus on the pan, place the raw bacon on top of the spears, and season with salt and pepper. Bake for 12 to 15 minutes, or until the bacon is almost crisp. Remove the pan from the oven and toss the bacon and asparagus. Crack the eggs over the top and bake until the eggs reach your desired doneness, about 5 to 7 minutes. Serve with the sliced avocado.

Makes 4 servings | **Prep time: 5 minutes** | **Cook time: 20 minutes**

NUT FREE, DAIRY FREE, GLUTEN FREE, PALEO, ONE PAN

12 uncured bacon slices

16 to 20 asparagus spears, ends snapped off and discarded

Salt

Freshly ground black pepper

8 large eggs

1 avocado, sliced

1. Preheat the oven to 425°F.

2. In large cast iron skillet over medium heat, cook the bacon. Turn the slices with tongs every few minutes and cook until the bacon is 75% cooked, 5 to 7 minutes. Transfer to a paper towel–lined plate.

3. Drain the bacon grease from the skillet and discard, leaving 3 tablespoons of bacon fat in the pan. Add the trimmed asparagus spears to the skillet, season with salt and pepper, and toss until coated with fat.

4. Bake in the oven for 6 to 8 minutes, or until the spears start to soften. Remove from the oven and turn the asparagus with tongs. Return the bacon to the skillet. Crack the eggs over the top of the bacon and asparagus.

5. Return the skillet to the oven and bake for 5 to 7 minutes, or until the eggs reach desired doneness.

6. Serve immediately with the avocado slices.

SUBSTITUTION TIP *Replace the asparagus with halved Brussels sprouts. Prepare them just like the asparagus, but the Brussels sprouts may need to bake for an additional few minutes before adding the bacon and eggs to the skillet. Another option would be adding halved cherry tomatoes prior to baking and topping the skillet with balsamic vinegar, fresh basil, and mozzarella cheese.*

. . . .

Per Serving Calories: 370; Total Fat: 27g; Saturated Fat: 8g, 66%; Protein: 23g, 25%; Total Carbs: 8g; Fiber: 5g; Net Carbs: 3g, 9%; Cholesterol: 394mg

Mexican Breakfast Bowl

You know those breakfast burritos that appear on just about every restaurant brunch menu these days? Well, here is the keto-friendly version in a bowl, with even more flavor and much fewer carbs. This is a super-filling dish that's also calorie dense, so make it the larger of your two main meals of the day.

Makes 2 servings | **Prep time: 10 minutes** | **Cook 10 minutes**

NUT FREE, GLUTEN FREE

1 tablespoon butter or ghee

1 cup cooked shredded pork

4 large eggs

2 tablespoons heavy
  whipping cream

Salt

Freshly ground black pepper

1 recipe Cauliflower "Rice"
  (page 118) (optional)

½ cup shredded Mexican
  blend cheese

1 avocado, pitted, peeled,
  and sliced

¼ cup sour cream

1 tablespoon chopped cilantro

1. In a skillet, melt the butter over medium-high heat. Add the pork and cook until it is crisped at the edges, about 5 minutes.

2. Meanwhile, in a small bowl, whisk the eggs and heavy cream, and season with salt and pepper.

3. If you are using the cauliflower "rice," divide it between two bowls.

4. When the pork is done crisping, remove it from the skillet and divide it between the two bowls. Push it to one half of the bowl, leaving room for the scrambled eggs.

5. Reduce the heat to medium, and scramble the eggs for 3 minutes or to your desired doneness.

6. Divide the eggs between the two bowls. Add the cheese, then the avocado slices, sour cream, and cilantro.

. . . .

Per Serving Calories: 680; Total Fat: 50.5g, 68%; Protein: 48.5g, 29%; Total Carbs: 9g; Fiber: 4.5g; Net Carbs: 4.5g, 3%

Cajun Cauliflower & Egg Hash

Although cauliflower is keto-friendly, many people complain that it's too bland to make it a diet staple. Not here! When combined with the intense flavors in this breakfast dish—think Cajun seasoning and pastrami scrambled with fresh eggs—the humble veggie truly shines.

Serves 4 | **Prep time: 10 minutes** | **Cook time: 20 minutes**

NUT FREE, DAIRY FREE, GLUTEN FREE, PALEO

1 (1-pound) bag frozen cauliflower florets

2 tablespoons extra-virgin olive oil

½ sweet yellow onion, chopped

4 large free-range eggs, lightly beaten

8 ounces shaved pastrami, chopped

½ green bell pepper, chopped

2 tablespoons minced garlic

1 teaspoon Cajun Seasoning

1. Set a steamer rack inside a large pot and pour in just enough water to come to the bottom of the rack. Bring the water to a boil over high heat. Add the cauliflower, cover the pot, and steam the cauliflower until tender, about 6 minutes. Drain the cauliflower and chop it into bite-size pieces. Set aside.

2. In a medium skillet, heat the olive oil over medium heat. Add the onion and sauté it until soft but not browned, 3 to 5 minutes.

3. Add the eggs to the skillet and gently stir to scramble them with the onion, about 2 minutes.

4. Stir the cauliflower, pastrami, green bell pepper, garlic, and Cajun seasoning into the scrambled eggs and onion. Continue cooking the mixture, stirring occasionally, until hot, about 5 minutes more. Serve immediately.

....

Per Serving Calories: 260; Total Fat: 15g; Saturated Fat: 4g, 54%; Protein: 22g, 36%; Total Carbs: 10g; Fiber: 4g; Net Carbs: 6g, 10%; Cholesterol: 225mg

Double Pork Frittata

Most frittatas are made with cheese, but this one uses heavy cream for the fluffiest, creamiest effect. Use all-natural pork lard if you can find it at your local butcher. That way, you can call this a triple pork frittata!

Serves 4 | **Prep time: 5 minutes** | **Cook 25 minutes**

NUT FREE, GLUTEN FREE

1 tablespoon pork lard or
  unsalted butter

8 large eggs

1 cup heavy (whipping) cream

Pink Himalayan salt

Freshly ground black pepper

4 ounces pancetta, chopped

2 ounces prosciutto, thinly sliced

1 tablespoon chopped fresh dill

1. Preheat the oven to 375°F. Coat a 9-by-13-inch baking pan with the lard or butter.

2. In a large bowl, whisk the eggs and cream together. Season with pink Himalayan salt and pepper, and whisk to blend.

3. Pour the egg mixture into the prepared pan. Sprinkle the pancetta in and distribute evenly throughout.

4. Tear off pieces of the prosciutto and place on top, then sprinkle with the dill.

5. Bake for about 25 minutes, or until the edges are golden and the eggs are just set.

6. Transfer to a rack to cool for 5 minutes.

7. Cut into 4 portions and serve hot.

COOKING TIP *You can use a greased muffin tin with this recipe to create individual egg bites. Just make sure to evenly distribute all the ingredients among the muffin cups.*

VARIATIONS *The great part about a frittata is that you can add so many other ingredients to it. Here are a few variations you can try, but have fun coming up with your own combinations from whatever is in your fridge:*

- *Browned sausage and fresh spinach*
- *Chopped bacon, sliced fresh mushrooms, and fresh spinach*
- *Sliced black olives, sliced red peppers, and chopped fresh parsley*
- *Diced ham, sliced green peppers, and sliced scallions*

Per Serving Calories: 437; Total Fat: 39g, 80%; Saturated Fat: 23g; Protein: 21g, 18%; Total Carbs: 3g, 2%; Fiber: 0g; Net Carbs: 3g; Cholesterol: 502mg

Mushroom Frittata

Frittatas can be described as baked omelets or as crustless quiches, but no matter what the description, they are delicious and simple. Any type of mushrooms can be used for the recipe, depending on what you like or what you have in your refrigerator. If you want to use portobello mushrooms, scoop out the black gills so that your eggs don't turn an unsightly gray.

Serves 6 | **Prep time: 10 minutes** | **Cook time: 15 minutes**

NUT FREE, GLUTEN FREE, ONE PAN

2 tablespoons olive oil

1 cup sliced fresh mushrooms

1 cup shredded spinach

6 bacon slices, cooked
  and chopped

10 large eggs, beaten

½ cup crumbled goat cheese

Sea salt

Freshly ground black pepper

1. Preheat the oven to 350°F.

2. Place a large ovenproof skillet over medium-high heat and add the olive oil.

3. Sauté the mushrooms until lightly browned, about 3 minutes.

4. Add the spinach and bacon and sauté until the greens are wilted, about 1 minute.

5. Add the eggs and cook, lifting the edges of the frittata with a spatula so uncooked egg flows underneath, for 3 to 4 minutes.

6. Sprinkle the top with the crumbled goat cheese and season lightly with salt and pepper.

7. Bake until set and lightly browned, about 15 minutes.

8. Remove the frittata from the oven, and let it stand for 5 minutes.

9. Cut into 6 wedges and serve immediately.

SUBSTITUTION TIP *If you're not keen on goat cheese, feta cheese tastes lovely with the other ingredients in this dish. Feta is higher in fat and lower in protein than goat cheese, so keep that in mind when considering your keto macros.*

. . . .

Per Serving Calories: 316; Total Fat: 27g, 80%; Protein: 16g, 16%; Total Carbs: 1g; Fiber: 0g; Net Carbs: 1g, 4%

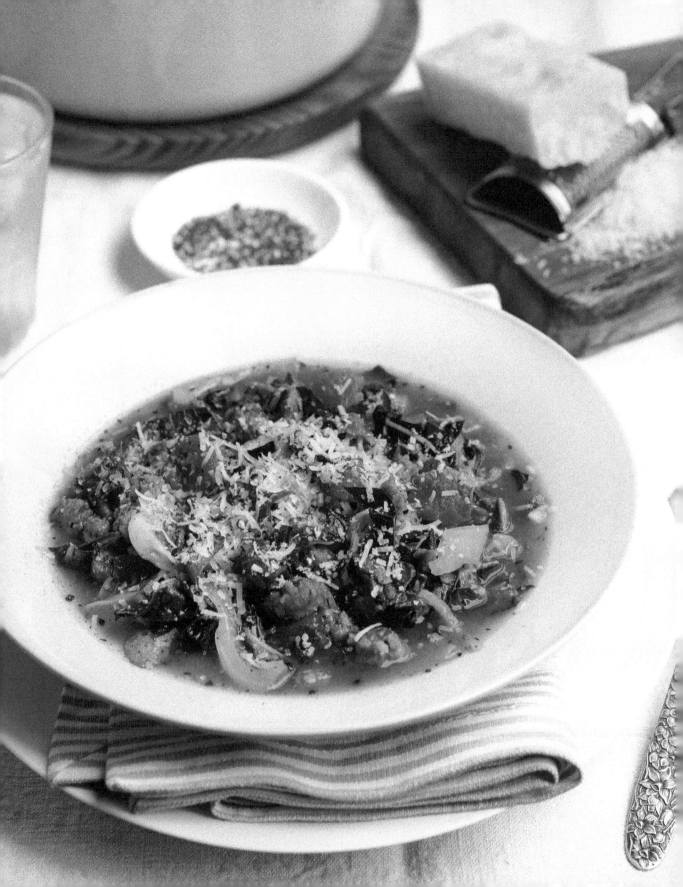

Soups
& Salads

....
Italian Sausage Soup, page 64

Creamy Tomato-Basil Soup

This soup is so fresh and creamy, you will never want to eat canned soup again. Serve it with a salad and Basic Bread (page 26) for a complete meal.

Serves 4 | **Prep time: 5 minutes** | **Cook 15 minutes**

VEGETARIAN, NUT FREE, GLUTEN FREE

1 (14.5-ounce) can diced tomatoes with Italian seasoning (such as Muir Glen)

2 ounces cream cheese

¼ cup heavy (whipping) cream

4 tablespoons unsalted butter

¼ cup chopped fresh basil leaves

Pink Himalayan salt

Freshly ground black pepper

1. Pour the tomatoes with their juices into a food processor (or blender) and purée until smooth.

2. In a medium saucepan over medium heat, cook the tomatoes, cream cheese, heavy cream, and butter for 10 minutes, stirring occasionally, until all is melted and thoroughly combined.

3. Add the basil, and season with pink Himalayan salt and pepper. Continue stirring for 5 minutes more, until completely smooth. If you wish, you could also use an immersion blender to make short work of smoothing the soup.

4. Pour the soup into four bowls and serve.

. . . .

Per Serving Calories: 239; Total Fat: 22g, 81%; Saturated Fat: 14g; Protein: 3g, 5%; Total Carbs: 9g, 14%; Fiber: 2g; Net Carbs: 7g; Cholesterol: 67mg

Cheesy Cauliflower Soup

Cauliflower can be used in seemingly anything. Soup is no exception. This is a keto take on a potato soup, minus all of those carbohydrates.

Serves 4 | **Prep time: 5 minutes** | **Cook 20 minutes**

NUT FREE, GLUTEN FREE, ONE PAN

1 tablespoon unsalted butter

½ onion, chopped

2 cups riced/shredded cauliflower (you can find riced cauliflower in your supermarket's produce section)

1 cup chicken broth

2 ounces cream cheese

1 cup heavy (whipping) cream

Pink Himalayan salt

Freshly ground pepper

½ cup shredded sharp Cheddar cheese

1. In a medium saucepan over medium heat, melt the butter. Add the onion and cook, stirring occasionally, until softened, about 5 minutes.

2. Add the cauliflower and chicken broth, and allow the mixture to come to a boil, stirring occasionally.

3. Lower the heat to medium-low and simmer until the cauliflower is soft enough to mash, about 10 minutes.

4. Add the cream cheese, and mash the mixture.

5. Add the cream and purée the mixture with an immersion blender (or you can pour the soup into the blender, blend it, and then pour it back into the pan and reheat it a bit).

6. Season the soup with pink Himalayan salt and pepper.

7. Pour the soup into four bowls, top each with the shredded Cheddar cheese, and serve.

SUBSTITUTION TIP *You could use cauliflower florets instead of riced cauliflower, but you will need to simmer the mixture longer before mashing it, 15 to 20 minutes. You could also use vegetable broth instead of chicken broth for a vegetarian soup.*

VARIATIONS *As with any creamy soup, crunchy ingredients added on top can be a perfect contrast:*
- *Top with crumbled bacon and chopped scallions along with the cheese.*
- *Add hot sauce for an extra kick.*

Per Serving Calories: 372; Total Fat: 35g, 84%; Saturated Fat: 4g; Protein: 9g, 8%; Total Carbs: 9g, 8%; Fiber: 3g; Net Carbs: 6g; Cholesterol: 108mg

Italian Sausage Soup

Soup is wonderful, especially in the fall and winter. This recipe makes a slightly spicy, comforting, and delicious Italian sausage soup that is the perfect cold-weather meal with a nice big salad on the side.

Makes 4 servings | **Prep time: 5 minutes** | **Cook 25 minutes**

NUT FREE, GLUTEN FREE, ONE PAN

1 tablespoon olive oil

½ onion, diced

3 garlic cloves, minced

8 ounces hot Italian sausage, removed from their casings

2 cups chicken broth

1 (14.5-ounce) can diced tomatoes

1 to 2 teaspoons red pepper flakes

1 teaspoon dried oregano

1 teaspoon dried basil

Salt

Freshly ground black pepper

¼ cup freshly grated Parmesan cheese, divided

2 cups chopped fresh spinach

1. In a large saucepan over medium heat, heat the olive oil.

2. Add the onion and garlic. Sauté for 5 to 7 minutes until the onion is softened and translucent.

3. Add the sausage to the pan. Cook for about 5 minutes as you crumble it, allowing the meat to brown.

4. Stir in the chicken broth and tomatoes. Bring to a boil and reduce the heat to low.

5. Add the red pepper flakes, oregano, and basil. Season with salt and pepper, and stir in 2 tablespoons of Parmesan. Simmer for 10 minutes and remove from the heat.

6. Stir in the spinach until wilted. Serve sprinkled with the remaining 2 tablespoons of Parmesan.

KALE VARIATION *Use kale instead of spinach—add it to the pan with the onion and garlic. Follow the rest of the recipe as written.*
CABBAGE VARIATION *Add ½ head cabbage, sliced, to the soup with the onion and garlic. You can do this with the original recipe or the kale variation (cabbage and kale together are delicious).*

....

Per Serving Calories: 365; Total Fat: 20g, 52%; Protein: 33g, 36%; Total Carbs: 11g; Fiber: 2g; Net Carbs: 9g, 12%; Sugar: 4g

Kale Variation Per Serving Calories: 377; Total Fat: 21g, 50%; Protein: 34g, 36%; Total Carbs: 14g; Fiber: 2g; Net Carbs: 12g, 16%; Sugar: 4g

Cabbage Variation Per Serving Calories: 397; Total Fat: 21g, 49%; Protein: 35g, 35%; Total Carbs: 17g; Fiber: 4g; Net Carbs: 13g, 16%; Sugar: 7g

Broccoli Cheddar Soup

A lot of soups like this one usually start with some butter and flour to thicken it up, but skipping the flour really doesn't make a difference, especially if you use heavy cream instead of regular milk. This soup is warm and nourishing and, more importantly, keto-friendly.

Serves 4 | **Prep time: 10 minutes** | **Cook time: 15 minutes**

NUT FREE, GLUTEN FREE, ONE PAN

4 tablespoons unsalted butter

1 celery stalk, diced

1 carrot, diced

½ onion, diced

1 garlic clove, minced

3 cups chicken broth

2 cups broccoli florets

1 cup heavy (whipping) cream

2½ cups shredded Cheddar cheese

Salt

Freshly ground black pepper

1. In a large saucepan over medium heat, melt the butter.

2. Add the celery, carrot, onion, and garlic. Stir to combine and sauté for 5 to 7 minutes until softened.

3. Stir in the chicken broth and bring to a simmer.

4. Add the broccoli. Simmer for 5 to 7 minutes then add the cream.

5. While stirring, slowly add the Cheddar, letting it melt completely. Season well with salt and pepper and serve hot. Refrigerate leftovers in an airtight container for up to 1 week.

BACON VARIATION *Top each serving with 2 crumbled pieces of cooked bacon.*

CHEESEBURGER VARIATION *Add 1 pound ground beef to the saucepan after the butter, celery, carrot, onion, and garlic. Cook for 7 to 10 minutes or until browned. Follow the rest of the recipe as written.*

. . . .

Per Serving Calories: 638; Total Fat: 58g, 80%; Protein: 23g, 15%; Total Carbs: 10g; Fiber: 2g; Net Carbs: 8g, 5%; Sugar: 3g

Bacon Variation Per Serving Calories: 721; Total Fat: 64g, 78%; Protein: 29g, 17%; Total Carbs: 10g; Fiber: 2g; Net Carbs: 8g, 5%; Sugar: 3g

Cheeseburger Variation Per Serving Calories: 856; Total Fat: 72g, 74%; Protein: 45g, 21%; Total Carbs: 10g; Fiber: 2g; Net Carbs: 8g, 5%; Sugar: 3g

Watercress-Spinach Soup

Watercress is a civilized green that is often used in fine dining as both an ingredient and a lovely garnish. The peppery, subtle taste of this plant is perfect with the more assertive spinach in this gorgeous soup. As its name implies, watercress grows in water, so its freshness is best maintained after purchase by submerging it back in water in a container in the refrigerator.

Serves 4 | **Prep time: 20 minutes** | **Cook time: 10 minutes**

NUT FREE, DAIRY FREE, GLUTEN FREE

2 tablespoons coconut oil

½ sweet onion, chopped

2 teaspoons minced garlic

1 tablespoon arrowroot

4 cups chicken stock

4 cups watercress

4 cups spinach

1 cup coconut milk

Sea salt

Freshly ground black pepper

8 cooked turkey bacon slices, chopped, for garnish

1. In a large saucepan over medium-high heat, heat the coconut oil. Sauté the onion and garlic in the oil until softened, about 3 minutes.

2. Whisk in the arrowroot to form a paste, then whisk in the chicken stock until the mixture is smooth. Add the watercress, spinach, and coconut milk.

3. Cook the soup until it is just heated through and the greens are still vibrant, about 3 minutes.

4. Transfer the soup to a food processor, and purée.

5. Transfer the soup back to the saucepan, and season with salt and pepper.

6. Top with the bacon, and serve.

....

Per Serving Calories: 280; Total Fat: 23g, 74%; Protein: 13g, 19%; Total Carbs: 7g; Fiber: 4g; Net Carbs: 3g, 7%; Sugar: 3g

Peanut-Chicken Soup

One-pot peanut soups are popular in West Africa and South America, where they can be as simple as shredded greens in a rich peanut broth or a thick, complex stew with meat, spices, and coconut milk, such as this version. The finished flavor of the soup will depend on the type and amount of curry paste you use. Green curry is quite mild, and if you crave true heat in your soup, try Thai red curry paste.

Serves 4 | Prep time: 10 minutes | Cook time: 15 minutes

DAIRY FREE, ONE POT

2 cups low-sodium chicken broth

1 cup coconut milk

½ cup natural peanut butter

2 tablespoons curry paste, or more if desired

1 cup diced tomatoes

1 cup shredded cooked chicken breast

1 teaspoon garlic powder

1 cup shredded spinach

1 tablespoon chopped fresh cilantro

1. In a large saucepan over medium-high heat, whisk together the chicken broth, coconut milk, peanut butter, and curry paste.

2. Bring the mixture to a boil, and reduce the heat to simmer for 4 minutes.

3. Stir in the tomatoes, chicken, and garlic powder, and simmer until the mixture is completely heated through, about 5 minutes.

4. Stir in the spinach and cilantro, and simmer until the greens are wilted, about 2 minutes.

5. Remove from the heat, and serve immediately.

....

Per Serving Calories: 471; Total Fat: 37g, 71%; Protein: 25g, 21%; Total Carbs: 14g; Fiber: 5g; Net Carbs: 9g, 8%; Sugar: 5g

Roasted Brussels Sprout Salad with Parmesan

The difference between this and most roasted Brussels sprouts dishes is that it calls for only the leaves of the sprouts, keeping it super light. Hazelnuts really play a starring role in this salad.

Serves 2 | **Prep time: 10 minutes** | **Cook 15 minutes**

VEGETARIAN, GLUTEN FREE

1 pound Brussels sprouts

1 tablespoon olive oil

Pink Himalayan salt

Freshly ground black pepper

¼ cup shaved or grated
   Parmesan cheese

¼ cup whole, skinless hazelnuts

1. Preheat the oven to 350°F. Line a baking sheet with a silicone baking mat or parchment paper.

2. Trim the bottom and core from each Brussels sprout with a small knife. This will release the leaves. (You can reserve the cores to roast later if you wish.)

3. Put the leaves in a medium bowl; you can use your hands to fully release all the leaves.

4. Toss the leaves with the olive oil and season with pink Himalayan salt and pepper.

5. Spread the leaves in a single layer on the baking sheet. Roast for 10 to 15 minutes, or until lightly browned and crisp.

6. Divide the roasted Brussels sprouts leaves between two bowls, top each with the shaved Parmesan cheese and hazelnuts, and serve.

SUBSTITUTION TIP *If you don't have hazelnuts, use chopped almonds.*

. . . .

Per Serving Calories: 297; Total Fat: 17g, 52%; Saturated Fat: 4g; Protein: 14g, 18%; Total Carbs: 22g, 30%; Fiber: 10g; Net Carbs: 13g' Cholesterol: 10mg

Blue Cheese & Bacon Kale Salad

Massaging the kale leaves with olive oil breaks down the fibers and makes the greens more tender and easier to digest. Top the kale with bacon, blue cheese crumbles, and pecans, and you have a nutritious salad packed with unique flavors and textures.

Serves 2 | **Prep time: 10 minutes** | **Cook 10 minutes**

GLUTEN FREE

4 bacon slices

2 cups stemmed and chopped fresh kale

1 tablespoon Herbed Balsamic Dressing (page 36), or your favorite vinaigrette dressing

Pinch pink Himalayan salt

Pinch freshly ground black pepper

¼ cup pecans

¼ cup blue cheese crumbles

1. In a medium skillet over medium-high heat, cook the bacon on both sides until crispy, about 8 minutes. Transfer the bacon to a paper towel–lined plate.

2. Meanwhile, in a large bowl, massage the kale with the vinaigrette for 2 minutes. Add the pink Himalayan salt and pepper. Let the kale sit while the bacon cooks, and it will get even softer.

3. Chop the bacon and pecans, and add them to the bowl. Sprinkle in the blue cheese.

4. Toss well to combine, portion onto two plates, and serve.

SUBSTITUTION TIP *Chopped almonds can replace the chopped pecans.*

. . . .

Per Serving Calories: 353; Total Fat: 29g, 74%; Saturated Fat: 9g; Protein: 16g, 16%; Total Carbs: 10g, 10%; Fiber: 3g; Net Carbs: 7g; Cholesterol: 52mg

Cobb Salad

Cobb salads make a great ketogenic meal. They are loaded with healthy fats and flavorful tidbits that make them much more than mere side salads. Having your protein and hardboiled eggs prepped will really cut down on your weeknight meal prep and is the key to quick recipes like this one. Serve this salad with Ranch Dressing (page 34) or your favorite low-carb bottled dressing.

Serves 4 | Prep time: 10 minutes

NUT FREE, GLUTEN FREE, ONE BOWL

4 cups chopped romaine lettuce

6 slices cooked bacon, crumbled

4 hardboiled eggs, peeled
  and sliced

2 cups cubed ham

1 cup crumbled blue cheese

2 avocados, sliced

1 cup cherry tomatoes, sliced

3 scallions, white and green
  parts, chopped

Ranch Dressing (page 34) or
  your favorite low-carb store
  bought dressing

Divide the lettuce evenly among 4 large salad bowls. Top each with the bacon, eggs, ham, cheese, avocados, tomatoes, and scallions, arranging the ingredients decoratively on top. Top with dressing and serve immediately.

SUBSTITUTION TIP *Don't stress if you don't have any ham in the fridge; you can use leftover chicken, shrimp, or another protein.*

....

Per Serving Calories: 529; Total Fat: 38g, 65%; Saturated Fat: 15g; Protein: 36g, 26%; Total Carbs: 12g, 9%; Fiber: 7g; Net Carbs: 5g; Cholesterol: 259mg

Flank Steak Salad

When in doubt, go for a salad! If it's one that's topped with flank steak, avocado, and feta cheese, you'll be glad you did. Salads are a great way to stay keto when dining out and are quick and easy to put together at home.

Makes 4 servings | **Prep time: 10 minutes** | **Cook time: 10 minutes**

NUT FREE, GLUTEN FREE, ONE PAN

¼ cup plus 2 tablespoons olive oil, divided

12 ounces flank steak

Salt

Freshly ground black pepper

6 cups fresh spinach

2 avocados, cubed

4 ounces feta cheese, crumbled

Juice of 1 lemon

1. Set the broiler to high.

2. Rub 2 tablespoons of olive oil all over the steak, and season on both sides with salt and pepper.

3. Place the steak on a broiler pan or sheet pan and cook under the broiler to your desired doneness (3 to 4 minutes per side for medium-rare).

4. Transfer the steak to a cutting board, and let it rest for 5 to 10 minutes.

5. While the steak is resting, in a salad bowl, toss together the spinach, avocado, and feta cheese. Add the remaining ¼ cup of olive oil and the lemon juice, season with salt and pepper, and toss to mix well. Divide the salad evenly among 4 serving bowls.

6. Slice the steak across the grain into thin strips, top each salad with one-quarter of the meat, and serve.

Per Serving Calories: 541; Total Fat: 46g, 75%; Saturated Fat: 9g; Protein: 24g, 16%; Total Carbs: 10g, 9%; Fiber: 7g; Net Carbs: 3g; Cholesterol: 25mg

Thai Shrimp & Zoodle Salad

Switch out your traditional greens with zoodles (zucchini noodles) in this salad for a fresh, crunchy twist! If you don't have your own spiralizer, you can buy pre-spiralized zoodles at your grocery store.

Serves 2 | **Prep time: 15 minutes** | **Cook time: 10 minutes**

NUT FREE, DAIRY FREE, GLUTEN FREE, PALEO

2 zucchini, spiralized (zoodles)

Salt

8 ounces peeled shrimp

¼ teaspoon paprika

2 tablespoons extra-virgin olive oil or ghee, divided

2 garlic cloves, minced

½ (15-ounce) can diced tomatoes with Italian seasoning (such as Muir Glen)

¼ teaspoon red pepper flakes

½ cup black olives, sliced

Freshly ground black pepper

¼ cup chopped fresh basil

1. Place the zoodles on a paper towel–lined plate and season with salt.

2. In a small bowl, season the shrimp with salt and the paprika.

3. In a skillet, heat 1 tablespoon of olive oil over medium-high heat. Add the shrimp and cook for about 2 minutes on each side. Set aside on a plate.

4. Reduce the heat to medium and add the remaining 1 table-spoon of olive oil. Cook the garlic until softened.

5. Add the tomatoes, red pepper flakes, and olives. Season with salt and pepper and heat until the mixture simmers.

6. Add the zoodles to the sauce and simmer for 2 minutes.

7. Add the shrimp and toss everything well.

8. Divide between two bowls and top with the basil.

Per Serving Calories: 335; Total Fat: 19g, 51%; Protein: 28g, 33%; Total Carbs: 13g; Fiber: 4g; Net Carbs: 9g, 16%

Bacon-Strawberry Spinach Salad

Berries are a keto-approved fruit, so you should aim to incorporate them into your diet a couple of times a week. It doesn't take a lot to add a refreshing sweetness, and just two strawberries really complement the fat in the bacon and avocado.

Serves 2 | **Prep time: 5 minutes** | **Cook time: 8 minutes**

NUT FREE, DAIRY FREE, GLUTEN FREE, PALEO

6 bacon slices

2 tablespoons extra-virgin olive oil

1 tablespoon freshly squeezed lemon juice

4 cups spinach

2 strawberries, sliced

1 avocado, pitted, peeled, and diced Salt

Freshly ground black pepper

1. In a large skillet over medium-high heat, cook the bacon on both sides until crispy, about 8 minutes. Transfer to a paper towel–lined plate to drain and cool, then crumble it.

2. In a small bowl, whisk together the olive oil and lemon juice.

3. In a large bowl, toss the spinach, bacon, strawberries, and avocado. Season with salt and pepper.

4. Drizzle the dressing on top and stir to combine. Serve.

Per Serving Calories: 380; Total Fat: 34g, 79%; Protein: 12g, 12%; Total Carbs: 10g; Fiber: 6g; Net Carbs: 4g, 9%

Chicken Salad

Chicken salad is easy to make in large quantities and use throughout the week. Since grapes are high-carb fruits, this recipe only calls for a few. For a satisfying lunch, scoop some of the salad into an avocado half, or serve with tender salad greens.

Serves 4 | Prep time: 10 minutes

NUT FREE, DAIRY FREE, GLUTEN FREE, ONE BOWL

1 (12.5-ounce) can
   chicken, drained
½ cup Keto Mayonnaise
   (page 30)
½ celery stalk, diced
1 scallion, green parts only,
   thinly sliced
½ cup grapes, finely diced
Salt
Freshly ground black pepper

In a large bowl, combine the chicken, mayonnaise, celery, scallion, and grapes. Season with salt and pepper and stir until combined. Serve immediately or refrigerate in an airtight container for up to 5 days.

CURRY VARIATION *Skip the grapes and add 1 tablespoon curry powder to the salad. Stir well.*
CUCUMBER DILL VARIATION *Add ½ cucumber, finely diced, and about 2 tablespoons chopped fresh dill to the chicken salad. Squeeze the juice of ½ lemon over everything and stir well to combine.*

. . . .

Per Serving Calories: 291; Total Fat: 17g, 52%; Protein: 23g, 33%; Total Carbs: 12g; Fiber: 0g; Net Carbs: 12g, 15%; Sugar: 5g

Curry Variation Per Serving Calories: 283; Total Fat: 17g, 54%; Protein: 23g, 34%; Total Carbs: 9g; Fiber: 1g; Net Carbs: 8g, 12%; Sugar: 2g

Cucumber Dill Variation Per Serving Calories: 297; Total Fat: 17g, 51%; Protein: 23g, 33%; Total Carbs: 13g; Fiber: 1g; Net Carbs: 12g, 16%; Sugar: 6g

Taco Salad

You can put this supper salad together on even the most hectic of weeknights, either for dinner or for lunch the next day. It's quick to prepare, and with cheese, sour cream, and avocado, it will fill you up and keep you satisfied.

Serves 4 | **Prep time: 10 minutes** | **Cook time: 15 minutes**

NUT FREE, GLUTEN FREE

1 tablespoon olive oil

½ white onion, diced

1 garlic clove, minced

1 pound ground beef

1 small packet taco seasoning
   (or 1½ teaspoons chili powder
   combined with 1½ teaspoons
   ground cumin)

Salt

Freshly ground black pepper

2 heads romaine
   lettuce, chopped

½ cup shredded Mexican
   blend cheese

¼ cup Pico de Gallo (page 31)
   or your favorite salsa

¼ cup sour cream

1 avocado, quartered and sliced

4 lime wedges

1. In a large saucepan over medium heat, heat the olive oil.

2. Add the onion and garlic. Sauté for 5 to 7 minutes until the onion is softened and translucent.

3. Add the ground beef and cook for 7 to 10 minutes until browned. Season with the taco seasoning, salt, and pepper. Drain and set aside.

4. Assemble the salads in four bowls: Start with lettuce. Top with seasoned ground beef. Sprinkle with cheese and add salsa, sour cream, and sliced avocado, and serve with a lime wedge.

CHICKEN VARIATION *Use shredded chicken instead of ground beef—cook 4 boneless skinless chicken breasts in a slow cooker (for 3 to 4 hours on high heat or 6 to 8 hours on low heat) with a jar of your favorite salsa. Shred with two forks and serve on the salads.*

....

Per Serving Calories: 597; Total Fat: 41g, 62%; Protein: 38g, 25%; Total Carbs: 19g; Fiber: 4g; Net Carbs: 15g, 13%; Sugar: 6g

Chicken Variation Per Serving Calories: 461; Total Fat: 25g, 50%; Protein: 36g, 30%; Total Carbs: 23g; Fiber: 5g; Net Carbs: 18g, 20%; Sugar: 8g

Asian Slaw

This is a great recipe for days when you feel like having Chinese food but don't want to spend much time cooking, and definitely don't want to stray from keto enough to order takeout! You will love the combination of napa cabbage with sesame oil, tangy vinegar, and crunchy almonds—and this recipe actually incorporates some veggies as well, so you get a little red bell pepper and sliced carrot. Enjoy it on its own, or toss in some shredded or chopped cooked chicken.

Serves 4 | Prep time: 15 minutes

VEGETARIAN, DAIRY FREE, GLUTEN FREE

1 head napa cabbage,
   thinly sliced

½ red bell pepper, julienned

½ carrot, julienned

¼ cup sliced almonds

¼ cup sesame oil

3 tablespoons rice wine vinegar

Juice of 1 lime

Salt

Freshly ground black pepper

1 teaspoon red pepper flakes

2 scallions, green parts
   only, sliced

2 tablespoons sesame seeds

Chopped fresh cilantro,
   for garnish

1. In a large bowl, combine the cabbage, bell pepper, carrot, and almonds.

2. In a small bowl, whisk together the sesame oil, vinegar, and lime juice. Season with salt and pepper. Stir in the red pepper flakes. Pour the dressing over the veggie mixture and toss well to combine.

3. Sprinkle with the scallions and sesame seeds. Toss again. Garnish with cilantro before serving.

PEANUT DRESSING VARIATION *Add 2 tablespoons unsweetened peanut butter to the dressing. Add 3 tablespoons crushed peanuts as a garnish along with the cilantro.*

AVOCADO VARIATION *Add 1 diced avocado for some extra fat.*

. . . .

Per Serving Calories: 229; Total Fat: 21g, 80%; Protein: 5g, 6%; Total Carbs: 8g; Fiber: 4g; Net Carbs: 4g, 14%; Sugar: 3g

Peanut Dressing Variation Per Serving Calories: 361; Total Fat: 32g, 77%; Protein: 11g, 10%; Total Carbs: 12g; Fiber: 5g; Net Carbs: 7g, 13%; Sugar: 4g

Avocado Variation Per Serving Calories: 320; Total Fat: 29g, 77%; Protein: 6g, 6%; Total Carbs: 14g; Fiber: 8g; Net Carbs: 6g, 17%; Sugar: 5g

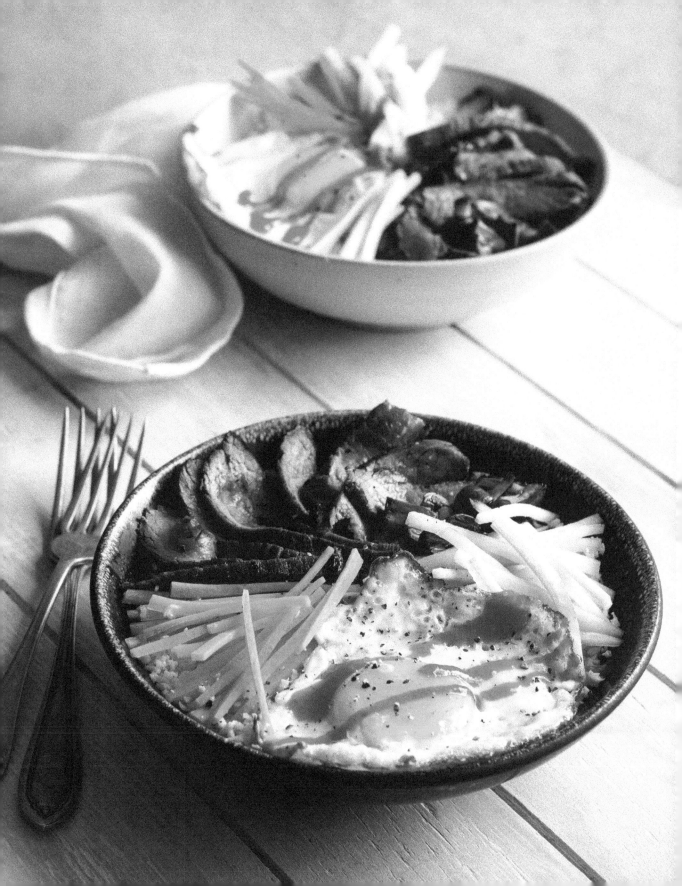

6

Lunch & Dinner

Steak & Egg Bibimbap, page 99

Zucchini Pesto Noodles

The scent of basil is always enticing. Here, it flavors a low-carb take on pesto pasta made with zucchini noodles. Go ahead and get creative with how you spiralize or slice your zucchini. As always, a good-quality sharp knife will make the job quick and easy.

Serves 4 | **Prep time: 10 minutes** | **Cook time: 10 minutes**

VEGETARIAN, GLUTEN FREE, ONE PAN

1 tablespoon olive oil

4 zucchini, cut or spiralized into noodles

2 tablespoons pesto, store-bought or homemade (page 32)

4 ounces cherry tomatoes (about 5 cherry tomatoes), halved

8 ounces small mozzarella balls, halved

6 basil leaves, chopped

Salt

Freshly ground black pepper

1. In a large skillet over medium heat, heat the olive oil. Add the zucchini noodles. Cook, stirring occasionally, for 3 to 4 minutes, until the zucchini is tender. Drain off any excess liquid.

2. Add the pesto, tomatoes, mozzarella, and basil, season with salt and pepper, and toss to mix. Cook for 2 to 3 minutes longer, until the cheese is melted. Serve immediately.

SUBSTITUTION TIP *Spaghetti squash can stand in for the zucchini as another healthy replacement for standard high-carb noodles. You don't even need a spiralizer or any special tool to prepare it. Halve the squash, scoop out the seeds, and bake it cut-side down at 425°F until tender, 30 minutes to an hour depending on the size. Once cooked and halved widthwise, the inside of the squash can be scraped with a fork, and the noodles appear like magic.*

....

Per Serving Calories: 221; Total Fat: 16g; Saturated Fat: 7g, 63%; Protein: 12g, 22%; Total Carbs: 8g; Fiber: 3g; Net Carbs: 5g, 15%; Cholesterol: 41mg

Cauliflower Steaks
with Bacon & Blue Cheese

This recipe is a heartier version of a classic wedge salad. Instead of lettuce, it has a warm, caramelized cauliflower steak as the base, which is topped with chunky blue cheese dressing and crispy bacon.

Serves 2 | **Prep time: 5 minutes** | **Cook time: 20 minutes**

NUT FREE, GLUTEN FREE, ONE PAN

½ head cauliflower

1 tablespoon olive oil

Pink Himalayan salt

Freshly ground black pepper

4 bacon slices

2 tablespoons blue cheese salad
   dressing

1. Preheat the oven to 425°F. Line a baking sheet with aluminum foil or a silicone baking mat.

2. To prep the cauliflower steaks, remove and discard the leaves and cut the cauliflower into 1-inch-thick slices. You can also roast the extra floret crumbles that fall off with the steaks.

3. Place the cauliflower steaks on the prepared baking sheet, and brush with the olive oil. You want the surface just lightly coated with the oil so it gets caramelized. Season with pink Himalayan salt and pepper. Place the bacon slices on the pan, along with the cauliflower floret crumbles.

4. Roast the cauliflower steaks for 20 minutes.

5. Place the cauliflower steaks on two plates. Drizzle with blue cheese dressing, top with crumbled bacon, and serve.

SUBSTITUTION TIP *You could follow the same instructions to make this dish with cabbage steaks instead of cauliflower.*

Per Serving Calories: 254; Total Fat: 19g, 68%; Saturated Fat: 9g; Protein: 11g, 16%; Total Carbs: 11g, 16%; Fiber: 4g; Net Carbs: 7g; Cholesterol: 47mg

Portobello Mushroom Pizza

What would pizza be without gooey melted mozzarella? Mozzarella is produced using a method that spins the cheese from milk and then cuts it, called pasta filata. Mozzarella is a good choice for the keto diet. It is high in fat (65 percent), contains about 32 percent protein, and has only 3 percent carbs. Enjoy them on their own as a light lunch, or pair them with grilled or broiled steak for dinner.

Serves 4 | **Prep time: 15 minutes** | **Cook time: 5 minutes**

VEGETARIAN, NUT FREE, GLUTEN FREE, ONE PAN

4 large portobello mushrooms, stems removed

¼ cup olive oil

1 teaspoon minced garlic

1 medium tomato, cut into 4 slices

2 teaspoons chopped fresh basil

1 cup shredded mozzarella cheese

1. Preheat the oven to broil. Line a baking sheet with aluminum foil and set aside.

2. In a small bowl, toss the mushroom caps with the olive oil until well coated. Use your fingertips to rub the oil in without breaking the mushrooms.

3. Place the mushrooms on the baking sheet gill-side down and broil the mushrooms until they are tender on the tops, about 2 minutes.

4. Flip the mushrooms over and broil 1 minute more.

5. Take the baking sheet out and spread the garlic over each mushroom, top each with a tomato slice, sprinkle with the basil, and top with the cheese.

6. Broil the mushrooms until the cheese is melted and bubbly, about 1 minute. Serve hot.

. . . .

Per Serving Calories: 251; Total Fat: 20g, 71%; Protein: 14g, 19%; Total Carbs: 7g; Fiber: 3g; Net Carbs: 4g, 10%

Crab Cakes

When working with crabmeat, fresh is best. Try to find large lump crabmeat. When incorporating crabmeat into your dish, fold it in gently during the final step of prep, and avoid overmixing.

Serves 4 | **Prep time: 10 minutes** | **Cook time: 10 minutes**

NUT FREE, DAIRY FREE, GLUTEN FREE, PALEO, ONE PAN

1 large egg

1 tablespoon freshly squeezed lemon juice

1 teaspoon Dijon mustard

3 tablespoons Keto Mayonnaise (page 30)

1 pound lump crabmeat

3 tablespoons coconut flour

Salt

Freshly ground black pepper

¼ cup coconut oil

1. In small bowl, whisk together the egg, lemon juice, mustard, and mayonnaise. Gently fold in the crabmeat, being careful not to break the crab up. Add the coconut flour, season with salt and pepper, and stir gently to combine.

2. Form the crab mixture into 8 patties.

3. In a large skillet over medium heat, melt the coconut oil. Cook the crab cakes for 3 to 5 minutes on each side. Serve immediately.

VARIATION TIP *For a little more heft and crunch, add ½ cup of crushed pork rinds to the crab cake mixture before cooking.*

Per Serving (2 patties) Calories: 498; Total Fat: 34g, 61%; Saturated Fat: 13g; Protein: 38g, 30%; Total Carbs: 10g, 9%; Fiber: 5g; Net Carbs: 5g; Cholesterol: 108mg

Baked Lemon-Butter Fish

Buttery, flaky fish goes perfectly with just about any side dish to make a healthy, keto-friendly meal. The lemon provides a bright counterpoint to the mild fish, and the capers give the dish a zesty pop.

Serves 2 | **Prep time: 10 minutes** | **Cook 20 minutes**

NUT FREE, GLUTEN FREE, PALEO

4 tablespoons unsalted butter, plus more for coating
2 (5-ounce) tilapia fillets
Pink Himalayan salt
Freshly ground black pepper
2 garlic cloves, minced
1 lemon, zested and juiced
2 tablespoons capers, rinsed and chopped

1. Preheat the oven to 400°F. Coat an 8-inch baking dish with butter.

2. Pat dry the tilapia with paper towels, and season on both sides with pink Himalayan salt and pepper. Place in the prepared baking dish.

3. In a medium skillet over medium heat, melt the butter. Add the garlic and cook for 3 to 5 minutes, until slightly browned but not burned.

4. Remove the garlic butter from the heat, and mix in the lemon zest and 2 tablespoons of lemon juice.

5. Pour the lemon-butter sauce over the fish, and sprinkle the capers around the baking pan.

6. Bake for 12 to 15 minutes, until the fish is just cooked through, and serve.

SUBSTITUTION TIP *You could use any mild white fish with this recipe. Even salmon is delicious with the lemon-butter sauce.*

Per Serving Calories: 299; Total Fat: 26g, 76%; Saturated Fat: 15g; Protein: 16g, 19%; Total Carbs: 5g, 5%; Fiber: 1g; Net Carbs: 3g; Cholesterol: 114mg

Creamy Dill Salmon

This salmon recipe is so easy and so creamy that you will love to make it for guests. Mayonnaise is a delicious way to create incredibly juicy fish or poultry and to get some healthy fats. And the fresh dill is the perfect herbal accent for salmon.

Serves 2 | **Prep time: 10 minutes** | **Cook 10 minutes**

NUT FREE, GLUTEN FREE, ONE PAN

2 tablespoons ghee, melted

2 (6-ounce) salmon
 fillets, skin on

Pink Himalayan salt

Freshly ground black pepper

¼ cup Keto Mayonnaise
 (page 30)

1 tablespoon Dijon mustard

2 tablespoons minced fresh dill

Pinch garlic powder

1. Preheat the oven to 450°F. Coat a 9-by-13-inch baking dish with the ghee.

2. Pat dry the salmon with paper towels, season on both sides with pink Himalayan salt and pepper, and place in the prepared baking dish.

3. In a small bowl, mix to combine the mayonnaise, mustard, dill, and garlic powder.

4. Slather the mayonnaise sauce on top of both salmon fillets so that it fully covers the tops.

5. Bake for 7 to 9 minutes, depending on how you like your salmon—7 minutes for medium-rare and 9 minutes for well-done—and serve.

INGREDIENT TIP *A lot of people might be unsure about eating the skin of the salmon, but a large amount of the healthy fats in salmon is found in the skin. Also, cooking the fish with the skin on helps retain moisture while cooking.*

. . . .

Per Serving Calories: 510; Total Fat: 41g, 72%; Saturated Fat: 11g; Protein: 33g, 26%; Total Carbs: 2g, 2%; Fiber: 1g; Net Carbs: 2g; Cholesterol: 114mg

Spicy Tuna Poke Bowl

Finding new ways to use avocado as a vessel for yummy flavors is always fun. In this recipe, avocado halves serve as the "bowls" for a Hawaiian-style raw tuna dish. The other great thing about this recipe is that raw fish means no cooking, so you can have this delicious meal ready in minutes!

Serves 2 | Prep time: 5 minutes, plus 20 minutes to marinate

NUT FREE, DAIRY FREE, GLUTEN FREE, PALEO

10 ounces sushi-grade ahi tuna, cubed

1 tablespoon sesame oil

1 tablespoon coconut aminos or soy sauce

1 tablespoon freshly squeezed lime juice

½ tablespoon lime zest

1 teaspoon peeled, grated fresh ginger

Freshly ground black pepper

1 tablespoon Keto Mayonnaise (page 30)

1 tablespoon Sriracha

2 avocados, halved and pitted

1 tablespoon sesame seeds or furikake

1 tablespoon chopped fresh chives

1. Rinse the tuna in cold water and pat dry. Cut into cubes and place in a medium mixing bowl.

2. In the same bowl, add the sesame oil, coconut aminos, lime juice, lime zest, and ginger. Season with pepper. Mix to coat and then place in the refrigerator for 10 to 20 minutes to marinate.

3. In a small bowl, mix the mayonnaise and Sriracha. If you like spice, you can add more Sriracha.

4. Remove the tuna from the refrigerator and spoon the mixture into the avocado halves.

5. Drizzle the Sriracha mayonnaise on top, and garnish with the sesame seeds and chives.

VARIATION *Traditionally, poke is served in a bowl with rice. If you prefer, you can cube the avocado and place all of the ingredients on top of a keto-friendly base, like fresh mixed greens, shirataki "rice," or cauliflower "rice."*

....

Per Serving Calories: 518; Total Fat: 34g, 59%; Saturated Fat: 8g; Protein: 37g, 29%; Total Carbs: 16g, 12%; Fiber: 10g; Net Carbs: 6g; Cholesterol: 44mg

Shrimp Scampi with Zoodles

Buttery, garlicky scampi always looks impressive on the table, yet you can whip it up in under 30 minutes, and there's very little prep work involved. This version uses zoodles (zucchini noodles) to keep it keto-friendly.

Serves 2 | **Prep time: 10 minutes** | **Cook time: 15 minutes**

NUT FREE, GLUTEN FREE

3 tablespoons unsalted
  butter or ghee

2 garlic cloves, minced

1 shallot, thinly sliced

12 ounces shrimp, peeled and
  deveined

¼ teaspoon red pepper flakes

½ lemon, juiced

1 tablespoon minced
  fresh parsley

2 zucchini, spiralized (zoodles)

Salt

Freshly ground black pepper

¼ cup grated Parmesan cheese

1. In a large skillet, melt the butter over medium heat. Add the garlic and shallot and sauté until softened.

2. In a small bowl, season the shrimp with the red pepper flakes and add to the skillet. Cook for about 1 minute and flip.

3. Once the second side is almost done, about 1 minute more, add the lemon juice. Reduce the heat slightly, then turn it off. Add the parsley and zoodles, and toss.

4. Season the scampi with salt and pepper. Divide between two plates and top with the Parmesan cheese.

VARIATION *Try adding veggies like cherry tomatoes, asparagus, or fresh spinach to your scampi. You can also add white wine at the same time as the lemon juice.*

. . . .

Per Serving Calories: 397; Total Fat: 24g, 52%; Protein: 40g, 43%; Total Carbs: 5g; Fiber: 0g; Net Carbs: 5g, 5%

Avocado Chicken Burgers

Possibly one of the simplest dinner recipes for the keto diet is an avocado chicken burger. Packed with healthy fats, avocado is the ultimate addition to any protein-based meal. Top these burgers with alfalfa sprouts and goat cheese or a slice of Swiss—however you serve them, they're a palate pleaser.

Serves 4 | **Prep time: 5 minutes** | **Cook time: 15 minutes**

DAIRY FREE, GLUTEN FREE

1 pound ground chicken

½ cup almond flour

2 garlic cloves, minced

1 teaspoon onion powder

¼ teaspoon salt

⅛ teaspoon freshly ground
   black pepper

1 avocado, diced

2 tablespoons olive oil

4 low-carb buns or lettuce wraps
   (optional)

1. In a large bowl, mix together the ground chicken, almond flour, garlic, onion powder, salt, and pepper.

2. Add the avocado, gently incorporating into the meat while forming four patties. Set aside.

3. In a large skillet over medium heat, heat the olive oil for about 1 minute. Add the patties to the skillet. Cook for about 8 minutes per side, or until golden brown and cooked through.

4. Serve on a low-carb bun, in a lettuce wrap (if using), or on its own.

INGREDIENT TIP *If using alfalfa sprouts, it's important to note that they can sometimes carry harmful bacteria. To avoid this problem, wash them a minimum of two times before consuming.*

. . . .

Per Serving (1 patty): Calories: 413; Total Fat: 25.7g, 57%; Saturated Fat: 5g; Protein: 33.9g, 32%; Total Carbs: 7.9g, 11%; Fiber: 5g; Net Carbs: 2.9g; Cholesterol: 96mg

Chicken-Basil Alfredo with Shirataki Noodles

You might find Miracle Noodles puzzling at first, because the cooking process for these noodles is different from what you are used to. But they can totally satisfy that pasta craving. This decadent "pasta" dish uses shirataki noodles, creamy Alfredo sauce, chicken, and fresh herbs. It is so filling and delicious!

Serves 2 | **Prep time: 10 minutes** | **Cook 15 minutes**

NUT FREE, GLUTEN FREE

FOR THE NOODLES
1 (7-ounce) package Miracle Noodle Fettuccini Shirataki Noodles

FOR THE SAUCE
1 tablespoon olive oil

4 ounces shredded cooked chicken (from a store-bought rotisserie chicken)

Pink Himalayan salt

Freshly ground black pepper

1 cup alfredo sauce (any brand you like)

¼ cup grated Parmesan cheese

2 tablespoons chopped fresh basil leaves

TO MAKE THE NOODLES

1. In a colander, rinse the noodles with cold water (shirataki noodles naturally have a smell, and rinsing with cold water will help remove this).

2. Fill a large saucepan with water and bring to a boil over high heat. Add the noodles and boil for 2 minutes. Drain.

3. Transfer the noodles to a large, dry skillet over medium-low heat to evaporate any moisture. Do not grease the skillet; it must be dry. Transfer the noodles to a plate; set aside.

TO MAKE THE SAUCE

1. In the saucepan over medium heat, heat the olive oil. Add the cooked chicken. Season with pink Himalayan salt and pepper.

2. Pour the Alfredo sauce over the chicken, and cook until warm. Season with more pink Himalayan salt and pepper.

3. Add the dried noodles to the sauce mixture, and toss until combined.

4. Divide the pasta between two plates, top each with the Parmesan cheese and chopped basil, and serve.

SUBSTITUTION TIP *To make this meal vegetarian, you need only replace the shredded chicken with sautéed mushrooms.*

Per Serving Calories: 673; Total Fat: 61g, 81%; Saturated Fat: 10g; Protein: 29g, 16%; Total Carbs: 4g, 3%; Fiber: 0g; Net Carbs: 4g; Cholesterol: 75mg

Chicken Piccata

An Italian restaurant classic gets the keto treatment in this dish. The unique flavor of the capers and lemon juice pairs well with the chicken and white wine. Traditionally made with chicken breast, this recipe calls for chicken thighs to increase the amount of fat.

Serves 4 | **Prep time: 10 minutes** | **Cook time: 15 minutes**

NUT FREE, DAIRY FREE, GLUTEN FREE

1 pound boneless chicken thighs

¼ teaspoon salt

⅛ teaspoon freshly ground black pepper

¼ cup olive oil

½ cup dry white wine

1 tablespoon freshly squeezed lemon juice

1 garlic clove, minced

1 tablespoon capers, chopped

3 tablespoons chopped fresh parsley

1. On a flat surface, flatten the chicken thighs with a meat tenderizer until they are ¼ inch thick. Season with the salt and pepper.

2. In a large skillet over medium heat, heat the olive oil for about 1 minute. Place two chicken thighs in the pan. Cook for about 4 minutes per side. Remove to a plate. Repeat, two at a time, with the remaining thighs. Set aside.

3. Using the same skillet, increase the heat to high. Add the white wine, lemon juice, garlic, and capers. Stir the sauce, scraping any browned bits from the bottom of the pan. Bring to a boil. Cook for 1 minute.

4. Add the chicken back into the pan. Heat in the sauce for 1 minute.

5. Add the parsley and stir to incorporate before serving.

. . . .

Per Serving Calories: 377; Total Fat: 29.7g, 74%; Saturated Fat: 7g; Protein: 20.3g, 24%; Total Carbs: 1.4g, 2%; Fiber: 0g; Net Carbs: 1.4g; Cholesterol: 95mg

Chicken Club Lettuce Wrap

This lettuce wrap is a great go-to meal when your only other option is the fast-food drive-through.

Serves 4 | Prep time: 5 minutes

NUT FREE, GLUTEN FREE, ONE BOWL

2 cups shredded cooked chicken (from 1 store-bought rotisserie chicken)

1 tomato, diced

1 avocado, sliced

6 slices cooked bacon, crumbled

4 tablespoons blue cheese crumbles

8 romaine lettuce leaves

Salt

Freshly ground black pepper

½ cup Ranch Dressing (page 34)

1. To prepare the lettuce wraps, divide the chicken, tomato, avocado, bacon, and cheese evenly among the lettuce leaves. Season with salt and pepper.

2. Drizzle ranch dressing over each lettuce wrap; serve cold.

Per Serving Calories: 405; Total Fat: 29g, 64%; Saturated Fat: 9g; Protein: 26g, 26%; Total Carbs: 9g, 10%; Fiber: 4g; Net Carbs: 5g; Cholesterol: 102mg

Sesame Pork & Green Beans

This dinner is quick and flavorful. It celebrates Asian flavors in a healthy and hearty dish that you can create in just minutes on a busy night.

Serves 2 | **Prep time: 5 minutes** | **Cook time: 10 minutes**

NUT FREE, DAIRY FREE

2 boneless pork chops

Pink Himalayan salt

Freshly ground black pepper

2 tablespoons toasted sesame oil, divided

2 tablespoons soy sauce

1 teaspoon Sriracha sauce

1 cup fresh green beans

Thinly sliced red chiles, for garnish

1. On a cutting board, pat the pork chops dry with a paper towel. Slice the chops into strips, and season with pink Himalayan salt and pepper.

2. In a large skillet over medium heat, heat 1 tablespoon of sesame oil.

3. Add the pork strips and cook them for 7 minutes, stirring occasionally.

4. In a small bowl, mix to combine the remaining 1 tablespoon of sesame oil, the soy sauce, and the Sriracha sauce. Pour into the skillet with the pork.

5. Add the green beans to the skillet, reduce the heat to medium-low, and simmer for 3 to 5 minutes.

6. Divide the pork, green beans, and sauce between two wide, shallow bowls and serve garnished with the red chiles.

SUBSTITUTION TIP *If Sriracha sauce is too spicy for you, you can add peeled, minced fresh ginger instead, which will add flavor and kick but not heat.*

. . . .

Per Serving Calories: 372; Total Fat: 25g, 60%; Saturated Fat: 7g; Protein: 35g, 36%; Total Carbs: 5g, 4%; Fiber: 2g; Net Carbs: 3g; Cholesterol: 55mg

Classic Roast Pork Tenderloin

Look out for sales at your grocery store, and buy a few packages of pork tenderloin to store in the freezer. Then, when you want to switch it up a bit or are on the verge of a particularly busy week, defrost it overnight in the refrigerator for this simple-yet-flavorful, five-ingredient main course.

Serves 4 | **Prep time: 5 minutes** | **Cook time: 25 minutes**

NUT FREE, DAIRY FREE, GLUTEN FREE, PALEO

2 tablespoons olive oil

1 (1½-pound) pork tenderloin

1 tablespoon Mrs. Dash Original Seasoning Blend or Trader Joe's 21 Seasoning Salute

Salt

Freshly ground black pepper

1. Preheat the oven to 425°F.

2. Drizzle the olive oil over the pork, sprinkle with the seasoning blend, and season with salt and pepper. Place the pork in a baking dish or on a baking sheet. Roast for 20 to 25 minutes or until the internal temperature reaches 145°F.

3. Refrigerate leftovers in an airtight container for up to 1 week.

PAN-SEARED VARIATION *If you have a little extra time, sear each side of the tenderloin in a skillet over the hotter side of medium-high heat with 1 tablespoon of olive oil. Just 2 to 3 minutes per side will give it some good color.*

SESAME ORANGE VARIATION *Brush the pork with a mixture of 2 tablespoons sesame oil, 1 tablespoon orange zest, and 1 teaspoon gluten-free soy sauce. Season with salt and pepper and follow the rest of the recipe as written.*

....

Per Serving Calories: 323; Total Fat: 20g, 54%; Protein: 35g, 46%; Total Carbs: 0g; Fiber: 0g; Net Carbs: 0g, 0%; Sugar: 0g

Pan-Seared Variation Per Serving Calories: 323; Total Fat: 20g, 54%; Protein: 35g, 46%; Total Carbs: 0g; Fiber: 0g; Net Carbs: 0g, 0%; Sugar: 0g

Sesame Orange Variation Per Serving Calories: 384; Total Fat: 26g, 61%; Protein: 35g, 39%; Total Carbs: 0g; Fiber: 0g; Net Carbs: 0g, 0%; Sugar: 0g

Herb & Dijon Pork Chops

Dijon mustard and Parmesan cheese add a delicious bite to these pork chops. Mixed with the mayonnaise, the creamy combination keeps the pork chops juicy and full of flavor.

Serves 2 │ **Prep time: 10 minutes** │ **Cook time: 17 minutes**

NUT FREE, GLUTEN FREE

1 tablespoon Dijon mustard

1 tablespoon Keto Mayonnaise (page 30)

½ teaspoon Italian seasoning

Salt

Freshly ground black pepper

2 boneless pork chops

¼ cup grated Parmesan cheese

1 teaspoon minced fresh parsley

1. Preheat the oven to 400°F.

2. In a bowl, mix the Dijon, mayonnaise, and Italian seasoning. Season with salt and pepper.

3. Pat the pork chops dry and season with salt and pepper. Place in a baking dish.

4. Spread the Dijon-mayonnaise mixture on the pork chops and sprinkle the Parmesan cheese on top.

5. Bake for 15 minutes. Adjust the oven to broil and cook for 1 to 2 minutes, until golden.

6. Remove the pork from the oven and let rest for 10 minutes. Sprinkle the parsley on top before serving.

VARIATION *The Dijon-mayonnaise mixture can also act as a marinade for the pork chops. Marinate for a few hours or even a full day. Then just sprinkle the Parmesan on before baking.*

....

Per Serving Calories: 323; Total Fat: 22g, 61%; Protein: 27g, 36%; Total Carbs: 3g, 3%; Fiber: 0g; Net Carbs: 3g

Walnut-Crusted Pork Chops

Pork chops are inexpensive, and with the right ketogenic "breading" (in this case, crushed walnuts and grated Parmesan cheese), you can take the flavor anywhere you want. Thick-cut pork chops work best because they stay juicy through the cooking process, but even with thin-cut chops you won't care about juiciness because you'll be enjoying so much more of the delicious coating. Serve this over zoodles for a great meal.

Serves 2 | Prep time: 10 minutes | Cook time: 20 minutes

GLUTEN FREE

3 tablespoons crushed walnuts

3 tablespoons grated
Parmesan cheese

Pinch sea salt

Pinch freshly ground
black pepper

1 large free-range egg

2 boneless free-range
pork chops

1. Preheat the oven to 400°F.

2. Line a rimmed baking sheet with parchment paper.

3. In a shallow dish, mix the walnuts, Parmesan cheese, salt, and pepper.

4. In another shallow dish, lightly beat the egg.

5. One at a time, dip a pork chop in the egg, coat it with the walnut and Parmesan mixture, and place it on the baking sheet.

6. Bake the chops for 10 minutes, flip them, and continue baking until they reach 145°F in the center, about 10 minutes more. Serve immediately.

....

Per Serving Calories: 352; Total Fat: 17g; Saturated Fat: 5g, 43%; Protein: 47g, 53%; Total Carbs: 2g; Fiber: 1g; Net Carbs: 1g, 4%; Cholesterol: 195mg

Steak, Mushroom & Pepper Kebabs

These are the best for summer cookouts—it's so easy to marinate some meat and veggies, skewer them, and take everything out to the grill. There are endless combinations of protein and veggies you can choose from, but these simple steak and mushroom kebabs are known crowd pleasers. Try serving them with a side of field greens and some Ranch Dressing (page 34) or a simple vinaigrette.

Serves 4 | Prep time: 15 minutes | Cook time: 15 minutes

NUT FREE, DAIRY FREE, GLUTEN FREE, PALEO

1 pound sirloin steak, cut into large cubes

8 ounces white button mushrooms or baby bella mushrooms

1 red bell pepper, seeded and cut into 1-inch squares

1 green bell pepper, seeded and cut into 1-inch squares

3 tablespoons extra-virgin olive oil

Salt

Freshly ground black pepper

1. Preheat the grill to medium-high heat.

2. In a large bowl, combine the cubed steak, mushrooms, and peppers. Add the olive oil and season with salt and pepper. Toss to combine. Alternate pieces of steak, mushroom, and pepper on metal skewers.

3. Grill for 6 to 8 minutes per side. Alternatively, cook the kebabs in a large skillet over medium-high heat. Remove from the heat, slide the steak and mushrooms from the skewers, and serve. Refrigerate leftovers in an airtight container for up to 5 days.

FAJITA VARIATION *Add ½ pound boneless skinless chicken breasts or thighs, cubed. Season with taco seasoning (or equal parts ground cumin and chili powder), salt, and pepper, and serve with lime wedges.*

. . . .

Per Serving Calories: 340; Total Fat: 24g, 67%; Protein: 27g, 35%; Total Carbs: 5g; Fiber: 1g; Net Carbs: 3g, 4%; Sugar: 2g

Fajita Variation Per Serving Calories: 416; Total Fat: 24g, 53%; Protein: 39g, 41%; Total Carbs: 9g; Fiber: 3g; Net Carbs: 7g, 8%; Sugar: 4g

Beef & Bell Pepper "Potato Skins"

In this low-carb version of a game day classic, big slices of bell pepper provide the "skin" to hold all the yummy ingredients while also offering a fresh, crisp taste. For additional flavor variations, add Mexican-inspired ingredients like diced onion, diced jalapeño or green chiles, chopped fresh cilantro, freshly squeezed lime juice (for the crema), or hot sauce.

Serves 2 | **Prep time: 10 minutes** | **Cook time: 20 minutes**

NUT FREE, GLUTEN FREE

1 tablespoon ghee

½ pound ground beef

Pink Himalayan salt

Freshly ground black pepper

3 large bell peppers, in different colors

½ cup shredded cheese (such as Mexican blend)

1 avocado

¼ cup sour cream

1. Preheat the oven to 400°F. Line a baking sheet with aluminum foil or a silicone baking mat.

2. In a large skillet over medium-high heat, melt the ghee. When the ghee is hot, add the ground beef and season with pink Himalayan salt and pepper. Stir occasionally with a wooden spoon, breaking up the beef chunks. Continue cooking until the beef is done, 7 to 10 minutes.

3. Meanwhile, cut the bell peppers to get your "potato skins" ready: Cut off the top of each pepper, slice it in half, and pull out the seeds and ribs. If the pepper is large, you can cut it into quarters; use your best judgment, with the goal of a potato skin–size "boat."

4. Place the bell peppers on the prepared baking sheet.

5. Spoon the ground beef into the peppers, sprinkle the cheese on top of each, and bake for 10 minutes.

6. Meanwhile, in a medium bowl, mix the avocado and sour cream to create an avocado crema. Mix until smooth.

6. When the peppers and beef are done baking, divide them between two plates, top each with the avocado crema, and serve.

SUBSTITUTION TIP *You could use ground turkey instead of ground beef.*

....

Per Serving Calories: 707; Total Fat: 52g, 66%; Saturated Fat: 17g; Protein: 40g, 22%; Total Carbs: 22g, 12%; Fiber: 10g; Net Carbs: 13g; Cholesterol: 136mg

Beef Stroganoff

Beef Stroganoff is the ultimate comfort food, and this keto-friendly version is no exception. Made with flavorful beef, butter, mushrooms, and sour cream, this dish will satisfy your cravings. In place of noodles, serve it over sautéed zucchini noodles or steamed spaghetti squash.

Serves 4 | **Prep time: 5 minutes** | **Cook time: 20 minutes**

NUT FREE, GLUTEN FREE, ONE PAN

1 pound ground beef

1 tablespoon salted butter

1 yellow onion, diced

2 cups mushrooms, sliced

2 garlic cloves, minced

1 cup beef broth

1 cup sour cream

¼ teaspoon xanthan gum

Salt

Freshly ground black pepper

Chopped fresh parsley, for
  garnish (optional)

Grated Parmesan cheese, for
  garnish (optional)

1. In a large skillet over medium-high heat, cook the ground beef, stirring and breaking it up with a spatula, until cooked through, 7 to 10 minutes. Drain the fat and transfer the meat to a paper towel–lined plate.

2. In the same skillet still over medium-high heat, melt the butter. Add the onion, mushrooms, and garlic and cook, stirring frequently, until the garlic is browned and the onion and mushrooms are tender, 5 to 7 minutes.

3. Add the broth, browned beef, sour cream, and xanthan gum to the skillet and cook, stirring, until the sauce is combined and thickened, 3 to 5 minutes.

4. Serve hot, garnished with the fresh parsley and grated Parmesan cheese (if using).

TIME-SAVER TIP *This recipe makes for great leftovers, freezes well, and can be paired with just about anything. After cooking, let it cool completely and store it in an airtight container in the refrigerator for 3 to 5 days or in the freezer for up to 3 months.*

Per Serving Calories: 369; Total Fat: 25g, 61%; Saturated Fat: 16g; Protein: 28g, 30%; Total Carbs: 8g, 9%; Fiber: 1g; Net Carbs: 7g; Cholesterol: 134mg

Steak & Egg Bibimbap

Bibimbap means "mixed rice" in Korean. While this recipe is unlike a traditional version, it has the key ingredients: beef, a runny egg, and vegetables. It's a great dish to make when you have leftover veggies in the fridge, because you can really throw in just about anything.

Serves 2 | **Prep time: 10 minutes** | **Cook time: 15 minutes**

NUT FREE

FOR THE STEAK

1 tablespoon ghee or
   unsalted butter
8 ounces skirt steak
Pink Himalayan salt
Freshly ground black pepper
1 tablespoon soy sauce or
   coconut aminos

FOR THE EGG
& CAULIFLOWER "RICE"

2 tablespoons ghee or unsalted
   butter, divided
2 large eggs
1 large cucumber, peeled and cut
   into matchsticks
1 tablespoon soy sauce
1 cup Cauliflower "Rice"
   (page 118)
Pink Himalayan salt
Freshly ground black pepper

TO MAKE THE STEAK

1. Using a paper towel, pat the steak dry. Season both sides with pink Himalayan salt and pepper.

2. Over high heat, heat a large skillet. Add the ghee or butter to the skillet. When it melts, put the steak in the skillet. Sear the steak for about 3 minutes on each side for medium-rare.

3. Transfer the steak to a cutting board and let it rest for at least 5 minutes.

4. Slice the skirt steak across the grain and divide it between two bowls.

TO MAKE THE EGG AND CAULIFLOWER "RICE"

1. In a second large skillet over medium-high heat, heat 1 tablespoon of ghee or butter. When the ghee is very hot, crack the eggs into it. When the whites have cooked through, after 2 to 3 minutes, carefully transfer the eggs to a plate.

2. In a small bowl, marinate the cucumber matchsticks in the soy sauce.

3. Clean out the skillet from the eggs, and add the remaining 1 tablespoon of ghee or butter to the pan over medium-high heat. Add the cauliflower "rice," season with pink Himalayan salt and pepper, and stir, cooking for 5 minutes. Turn the heat up to high at the end of the cooking to get a nice crisp on the "rice."

Continued

4. Divide the "rice" between two bowls.

5. Top the "rice" in each bowl with an egg, the steak, and the marinated cucumber matchsticks and serve.

SUBSTITUTION TIP *You could also make this recipe with ground turkey or beef instead of steak.*

VARIATIONS *You can add so many vegetables and other ingredients to a bibimbap, so take a look in your fridge and get creative. Delicious add-ins include:*
- *Kimchi*
- *Sriracha, drizzled on top*
- *Bean sprouts*
- *Carrot matchsticks*
- *Chopped mushrooms*
- *Chopped scallions*

. . . .

Per Serving Calories: 590; Total Fat: 45g, 68%; Saturated Fat: 18g; Protein: 39g, 26%; Total Carbs: 8g, 6%; Fiber: 4g; Net Carbs: 5g; Cholesterol: 280mg

Keto Chicken-Fried Steak

Crispy chicken-fried steak gets a keto makeover in this recipe with ground pork rinds and coconut flour. Make sure you get the oil nice and hot before adding the dredged steak—you want it to really sizzle so it gets perfectly crispy.

Serves 2 | **Prep time: 15 minutes** | **Cook time: 10 minutes**

NUT FREE, DAIRY FREE, GLUTEN FREE, PALEO

½ pound cube steak

1 large egg

½ cup coconut flour

1 teaspoon cayenne pepper

Salt

Freshly ground black pepper

½ cup ground pork rinds

¼ cup extra-virgin olive oil, or enough to coat the bottom of the skillet

1. Using a mallet, pound the cube steak to tenderize it.

2. In a shallow bowl, lightly beat the egg. On a large plate, mix the coconut flour and cayenne pepper. Season with salt and pepper. On another large plate, add the pork rind "bread" crumbs.

3. Dredge the steak on both sides in the coconut flour mixture. Dip into the egg, coating both sides. Dredge in the pork rind crumbs, pressing the pork rinds into the steak so they stick.

4. In a large skillet, heat the olive oil over medium-high heat until the oil sizzles. Cook the "breaded" steak for 4 minutes per side, flipping once, until golden and crispy.

VARIATION *You can add additional seasoning to the "breading" by using flavored pork rinds or adding Mexican Spice Blend (page 38).*

. . . .

Per Serving Calories: 485; Total Fat: 30g, 56%; Saturated Fat: 10g; Protein: 34g, 28%; Total Carbs: 19g, 16%; Fiber: 12g; Net Carbs: 7g; Cholesterol: 65mg

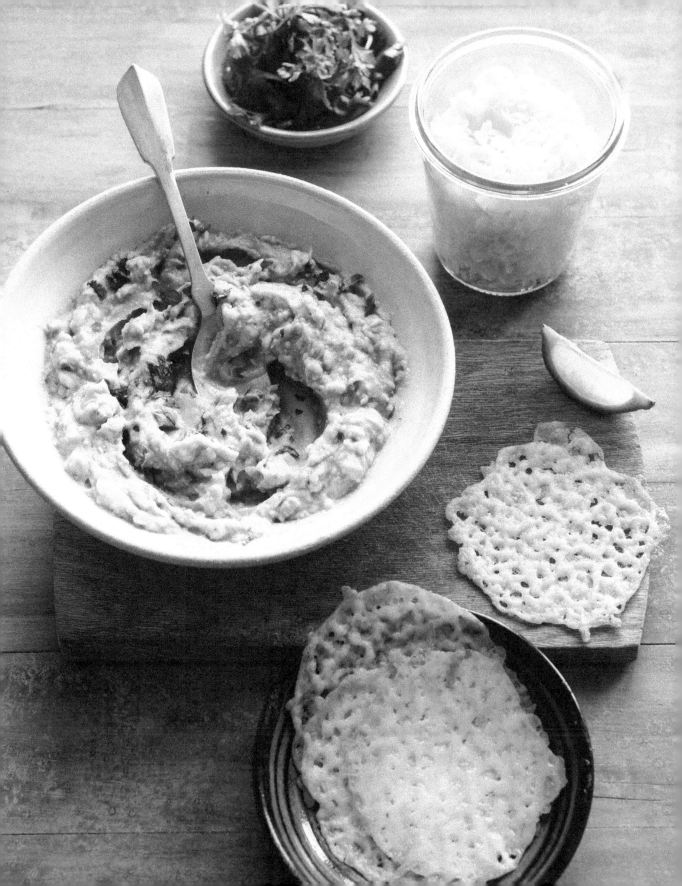

7

Snacks

Cheese Chips & Guacamole, page 111

Rosemary Roasted Almonds

Fresh rosemary is key here, so save this recipe for another time if you only have dried rosemary on hand. Enjoy these nuts with a cup of tea or alongside cured meats and cheeses.

Serves 4 | **Prep time: 5 minutes** | **Cook time: 15 minutes**

VEGETARIAN, DAIRY FREE, GLUTEN FREE

1½ cups almonds

1 tablespoon olive oil

1 tablespoon chopped fresh
  rosemary

½ teaspoon salt

½ teaspoon freshly ground
  black pepper

¼ teaspoon ground ginger

1. Preheat the oven to 325°F.

2. In a medium bowl, combine the almonds and olive oil. Mix until the almonds are evenly coated.

3. Add the rosemary, salt, pepper, and ginger to the almonds. Stir to combine.

4. On a baking sheet covered with aluminum foil, spread the almonds into an even layer. Place the sheet in the preheated oven. Bake for 15 minutes, or until toasted.

INGREDIENT TIP *Almonds are often less expensive per pound when purchased in bulk. Look for bulk dry goods sections at your grocery store or visit a store like Costco for the best deals.*

. . . .

Per Serving (½ cup) Calories: 253; Total Fat: 21g, 74%; Saturated Fat: 2g; Protein: 8g, 13%; Total Carbs: 8g, 13%; Fiber: 5g; Net Carbs: 3g; Cholesterol: 0mg

Herb & Walnut–Crusted Goat Cheese

Goat cheese is a marvelous tart creation that has about 12 grams of fat, 10 grams of protein, and zero carbs in a 2-ounce portion, which is the recommended serving size in this recipe. Try to find soft goat cheese because semi-hard and hard types actually do contain carbs. The soft product can be found in most grocery stores in prepackaged logs.

Serves 4 | Prep time: 10 minutes

VEGETARIAN, GLUTEN FREE

6 ounces chopped walnuts

1 tablespoon chopped oregano

1 tablespoon chopped parsley

1 teaspoon chopped fresh thyme

¼ teaspoon freshly ground
   black pepper

1 (8-ounce) log goat cheese

1. Place the walnuts, oregano, parsley, thyme, and pepper in a food processor and pulse until finely chopped.

2. Pour the walnut mixture onto a plate and roll the goat cheese log in the nut mixture, pressing so the cheese is covered and the walnut mixture sticks to the log.

3. Wrap the cheese in plastic and store in the refrigerator for up to 1 week. Slice and enjoy!

. . . .

Per Serving Calories: 304; Total Fat: 28g, 77%; Protein: 12g, 18%; Total Carbs: 4g; Fiber: 2g; Net Carbs: 2g, 6%

Seaweed Square Pileups

Seaweed squares are great on their own for snacking, but they also present the perfect canvas to create quick pile ups with sushi-inspired ingredients. Once you make this recipe, experiment with topping combinations of your own. Imagine anything you find in sushi, like cucumbers and crab, and go from there.

Serves 2 | Prep time: 10 minutes

VEGETARIAN, NUT FREE, DAIRY FREE, PALEO

6 seaweed snack squares

4 ounces smoked salmon

½ avocado, pitted

1 teaspoon soy sauce or coconut aminos

1 tablespoon Everything Seasoning (page 37)

1. On a work surface, lay out the seaweed snack squares in a single layer. Divide the salmon evenly between the seaweed squares.

2. Using a fork, scrape the flesh from the avocado, transfer to a small bowl, and mash it. Mix in the soy sauce. Place a dollop of the avocado on top of each square. Sprinkle the everything seasoning on top. To eat, fold like a taco and enjoy.

. . . .

Per Serving Calories: 165; Total Fat: 9g, 45%; Protein: 19g, 40%; Total Carbs: 6g; Fiber: 3g; Net Carbs: 3g, 15%

Cucumber Bites

Cucumbers are a great vehicle for flavors. Here, they are used as shot glasses. Sounds fun, right? It is! Fill them up with dairy-free cream cheese and any other flavor combinations you can dream up.

Serves 2 | **Prep time: 10 minutes**

DAIRY FREE, PALEO

1 cucumber

Salt

2 tablespoons dairy-free cream cheese

1 cooked bacon slice, crumbled

½ jalapeño pepper, diced fine

1. Cut the cucumber into 1-inch slices and scoop the seeds out of the top to create a cup (or shot glass as I like to call it). I peel my cucumber, but you don't have to. Season with salt.

2. In a small bowl, mix the dairy-free cream cheese with the crumbled bacon and jalapeño pepper. Spoon the mixture into the cucumber cups.

VARIATION *Dill and little bits of smoked salmon is another yummy combination.*

....

Per Serving Calories: 95; Total Fat: 7g, 68%; Saturated Fat: 4g; Protein: 3g, 11%; Total Carbs: 6g, 21%; Fiber: 1g; Net Carbs: 5g; Cholesterol: 21mg

Bacon-Cheese Deviled Eggs

A simple favorite is made extra special with the addition of bacon and tasty Swiss cheese. Eggs are a wonderful addition to the keto diet because they are an excellent source of fat and protein, about 63 percent and 35 percent, respectively, in one large egg. Deviled eggs can be eaten as a quick snack or taken to a get-together on a pretty platter for everyone to enjoy.

Serves 12 │ **Prep time: 15 minutes**

NUT FREE, GLUTEN FREE

6 large eggs, hardboiled
 and peeled
¼ cup Keto Mayonnaise
 (page 30)
¼ avocado, chopped
¼ cup Swiss cheese, finely
 shredded
½ teaspoon Dijon mustard
Freshly ground black pepper
6 bacon slices, cooked
 and chopped

1. Halve each of the eggs lengthwise.

2. Carefully remove the yolk and place the yolks in a medium bowl. Place the whites, hollow-side up, on a plate.

3. Mash the yolks with a fork and add the mayonnaise, avocado, cheese, and Dijon mustard. Stir until well mixed. Season the yolk mixture with the black pepper.

4. Spoon the yolk mixture back into the egg white hollows and top each egg half with the chopped bacon.

5. Store the eggs in an airtight container in the refrigerator for up to 1 day.

TIME-SAVING TIP *Hardboiled eggs make perfect snacks and a great addition to many recipes such as salads and entrees. Hard-boil a dozen eggs at the beginning of the week and keep them in the refrigerator for when you need them.*

Per Serving (1 deviled egg) Calories: 85; Total Fat: 7g, 70%; Protein: 6g, 25%; Total Carbs: 2g; Fiber: 0g; Net Carbs: 2g, 5%

Keto Spinach & Artichoke Dip

This is the easiest way to make one of the most popular party dips out there. It's great on its own, on top of chicken, or with sliced veggies for dipping instead of the more traditional high-carb toast or crackers.

Serves 6 | **Prep time: 5 minutes** | **Cook time: 10 minutes**

VEGETARIAN, NUT FREE, GLUTEN FREE

1 cup frozen chopped spinach, thawed and drained

1½ cups canned artichoke hearts, drained and chopped

Salt

Freshly ground black pepper

8 ounces cream cheese

¼ cup sour cream

¼ cup Keto Mayonnaise (page 30)

⅓ cup grated Parmesan cheese

1 teaspoon garlic powder

1 teaspoon red pepper flakes

1. In a small saucepan over medium-low heat, combine the spinach and artichokes. Season with salt and pepper.

2. Add the cream cheese and stir to combine until completely melted. Remove from the heat and stir in the sour cream, mayonnaise, Parmesan, garlic powder, and red pepper flakes. Serve hot.

BAKED VARIATION *Mix together all the ingredients in an 8- or 9-inch square baking dish and top with ¼ cup shredded mozzarella. Bake at 350°F for 20 minutes or until the cheese melts.*

SLOW COOKER VARIATION *If you want to make a double batch ahead of time, mix everything together and cook in your slow cooker on low heat for 2 hours.*

. . . .

Per Serving Calories: 223; Total Fat: 20g, 80%; Protein: 6g, 10%; Total Carbs: 7g; Fiber: 1g; Net Carbs: 6g, 10%; Sugar: 2g

Baked Variation Per Serving Calories: 223; Total Fat: 20g, 80%; Protein: 6g, 10%; Total Carbs: 7g; Fiber: 1g; Net Carbs: 6g, 10%; Sugar: 2g

Slow Cooker Variation Per Serving Calories: 223; Total Fat: 20g, 80%; Protein: 6g, 10%; Total Carbs: 7g; Fiber: 1g; Net Carbs: 6g, 10%; Sugar: 2g

Queso Dip

Also known as *chile con queso*, this dip originated in Mexico and can be found in many places that serve Tex-Mex cuisine. Jalapeño peppers are hot because they contain capsaicin. They are considered about medium in heat on the Scoville scale, with about 2,500 to 8,000 heat units per pepper. If you want a hotter dip, choose a pepper with more heat units, such as a habanero or Scotch bonnet chile. Drizzle this over Taco Salad (page 75) or serve it with keto crackers or low-carb veggies.

Serves 6 | **Prep time: 5 minutes** | **Cook time: 10 minutes**

VEGETARIAN, NUT FREE, GLUTEN FREE, ONE POT

½ cup coconut milk

½ jalapeño pepper, seeded and diced

1 teaspoon minced garlic

½ teaspoon onion powder

2 ounces goat cheese

6 ounces sharp Cheddar cheese, shredded

¼ teaspoon cayenne pepper

1. Place a medium pot over medium heat and add the coconut milk, jalapeño, garlic, and onion powder.

2. Bring the liquid to a simmer and then whisk in the goat cheese until smooth.

3. Add the Cheddar cheese and cayenne and whisk until the dip is thick, 30 seconds to 1 minute.

4. Pour into a serving dish and serve with keto crackers or low-carb vegetables.

....

Per Serving Calories: 213; Total Fat: 19g, 79%; Protein: 10g, 19%; Total Carbs: 2g; Fiber: 0g; Net Carbs: 2g, 2%

Cheese Chips & Guacamole

Chips and guacamole is one of those appetizers you miss when you are on a keto diet. But these cheese chips are so easy to make, there is no reason to miss chips. And you may even like these better! For an extra kick, add some of the diced jalapeños to the cheese mixture before baking the chips.

Serves 2 | **Prep time: 10 minutes** | **Cook time: 10 minutes**

VEGETARIAN, NUT FREE, GLUTEN FREE

FOR THE CHEESE CHIPS

1 cup shredded cheese (such as Mexican blend)

FOR THE GUACAMOLE

1 avocado, mashed

Juice of ½ lime

1 teaspoon diced jalapeño

2 tablespoons chopped fresh cilantro leaves

Pink Himalayan salt

Freshly ground black pepper

TO MAKE THE CHEESE CHIPS

1. Preheat the oven to 350°F. Line a baking sheet with parchment paper or a silicone baking mat.

2. Add ¼-cup mounds of shredded cheese to the pan, leaving plenty of space between them, and bake until the edges are brown and the middles have fully melted, about 7 minutes.

3. Set the pan on a cooling rack, and let the cheese chips cool for 5 minutes. The chips will be floppy when they first come out of the oven but will crisp as they cool.

TO MAKE THE GUACAMOLE

1. In a medium bowl, mix together the avocado, lime juice, jalapeño, and cilantro, and season with pink Himalayan salt and pepper.

2. Top the cheese chips with the guacamole, and serve.

. . . .

Per Serving Calories: 323; Total Fat: 27g, 75%; Saturated Fat: 14g; Protein: 15g, 16%; Total Carbs: 8g, 9%; Fiber: 5g; Net Carbs: 3g; Cholesterol: 59mg

Cheesy Spinach Puffs

These little cheesy spinach balls are a great keto appetizer to bring to your next potluck to make sure there's at least one thing you can eat (although there's usually a charcuterie or cheese board around somewhere, which is all you really need).

Serves 6 to 8 | **Prep time: 10 minutes** | **Cook time: 10 minutes** | **Chill time: 10 minutes**

VEGETARIAN, GLUTEN FREE

16 ounces frozen spinach, thawed, drained, and squeezed of as much excess liquid as possible

1 cup almond flour

4 tablespoons butter, melted, plus more for the baking sheet

2 eggs

¼ cup grated Parmesan cheese

¼ cup cream cheese

3 tablespoons heavy (whipping) cream

1 tablespoon onion powder

1 teaspoon garlic powder

Salt

Freshly ground black pepper

1. In a food processor, combine the spinach, almond flour, butter, eggs, Parmesan, cream cheese, cream, onion powder, and garlic powder. Season with salt and pepper. Blend until smooth. Transfer to the refrigerator and chill for 10 to 15 minutes.

2. Preheat the oven to 350°F.

3. Grease a baking sheet with butter.

4. Scoop the spinach mixture in heaping tablespoons and roll into balls. Place on the prepared baking sheet and bake for about 10 minutes until set. When tapped with your finger, they should not still be soft. Enjoy warm (best!) or cold. Refrigerate in an airtight container for up to 4 days.

FETA VARIATION *Use feta instead of cream cheese.*
BACON VARIATION *Top these puffs with crumbled cooked bacon.*

. . . .

Per Serving Calories: 159; Total Fat: 14g, 78%; Protein: 6g, 14%; Total Carbs: 3g; Fiber: 2g; Net Carbs: 1g, 8%; Sugar: 1g

Feta Variation Per Serving Calories: 147; Total Fat: 13g, 76%; Protein: 6g, 15%; Total Carbs: 3g; Fiber: 2g; Net Carbs: 1g, 9%; Sugar: 1g

Bacon Variation Per Serving Calories: 200; Total Fat: 17g, 76%; Protein: 9g, 17%; Total Carbs: 3g; Fiber: 2g; Net Carbs: 1g, 7%; Sugar: 1g

Bacon-Wrapped Jalapeños

These game-day snacks are so easy to make, with only three ingredients, but the prep time can be a killer if you don't use gloves to keep the hot pepper juices off your hands (see Ingredient Tip). Make an extra batch on Sunday, and enjoy them throughout the week.

Serves 4 | **Prep time: 10 minutes** | **Cook time: 20 minutes**

NUT FREE, GLUTEN FREE, ONE PAN

10 jalapeños

8 ounces cream cheese, at room temperature

1 pound bacon (you will use about half a slice per popper)

1. Preheat the oven to 450°F. Line a baking sheet with aluminum foil or a silicone baking mat.

2. Halve the jalapeños lengthwise, and remove the seeds and membranes (if you like the extra heat, leave them in). Place them on the prepared pan cut-side up.

3. Spread some of the cream cheese inside each jalapeño half.

4. Wrap a jalapeño half with a slice of bacon (depending on the size of the jalapeño, use a whole slice of bacon, or half).

5. Secure the bacon around each jalapeño with 1 to 2 toothpicks so it stays put while baking.

6. Bake for 20 minutes, until the bacon is done and crispy. Serve hot or at room temperature.

INGREDIENT TIP *I recommend wearing thin rubber gloves when you are prepping a batch of fresh jalapeños. The capsaicin from chiles soaks into your skin, and even after washing your hands multiple times, it can still be irritating. It is so easy to forget and touch your eyes or face.*

Per Serving Calories: 721; Total Fat: 70g, 87%; Saturated Fat: 28g; Protein: 17g, 10%; Total Carbs: 5g, 3%; Fiber: 1g; Net Carbs: 4g; Cholesterol: 139mg

Avocado Fries

These avocado fries are breaded in almond flour and actually get a little crispy in the oven, which can be a welcome change when you're eating a keto diet. Serve them as a side with almost anything in the Lunch & Dinner chapter of this book.

Serves 2 | Prep time: 10 minutes | Cook time: 20 minutes

VEGETARIAN, DAIRY FREE, GLUTEN FREE

Nonstick olive oil cooking spray, or olive oil

1 cup almond flour

¼ teaspoon garlic powder

¼ teaspoon onion powder

Salt

Freshly ground black pepper

1 egg

2 large avocados, halved and pitted, each half cut into 4 or 5 slices

Chipotle Aioli, for dipping (optional; recipe follows)

1. Preheat the oven to 425°F. Spray a baking sheet with olive oil spray or coat with a little olive oil.

2. Place the almond flour in a shallow dish and season it with the garlic powder, onion powder, and some salt and pepper.

3. In another shallow dish, whisk the egg.

4. Dip both sides of each avocado slice first into the egg and then into the seasoned almond flour. Cover both sides with the flour and place on the prepared baking sheet. Spray the fries with a fine mist of cooking spray.

5. Bake for 15 to 20 minutes or until the almond flour browns slightly. Remove from the oven and serve immediately.

CHIPOTLE AIOLI VARIATION *In a blender, mix ½ cup Keto Mayonnaise (page 30) with 2 canned chiles in adobo sauce. Season with salt and pepper and serve as a dipping sauce for the avocado fries.*

PAN-FRIED VARIATION *Brown the avocado fries in a skillet instead of the oven: use about 1 tablespoon olive oil and cook over medium-high heat for 2 to 3 minutes per side.*

....

Per Serving Calories: 436; Total Fat: 36g, 74%; Protein: 9g, 9%; Total Carbs: 19g; Fiber: 13g; Net Carbs: 6g, 17%; Sugar: 1g

Chipotle Aioli Per Serving Calories: 723; Total Fat: 67g, 83%; Protein: 11g, 6%; Total Carbs: 19g; Fiber: 14g; Net Carbs: 5g, 11%; Sugar: 1g

Pan-Fried Per Serving Calories: 490; Total Fat: 42g, 77%; Protein: 9g, 8%; Total Carbs: 19g; Fiber: 13g; Net Carbs: 6g, 16%; Sugar: 1g

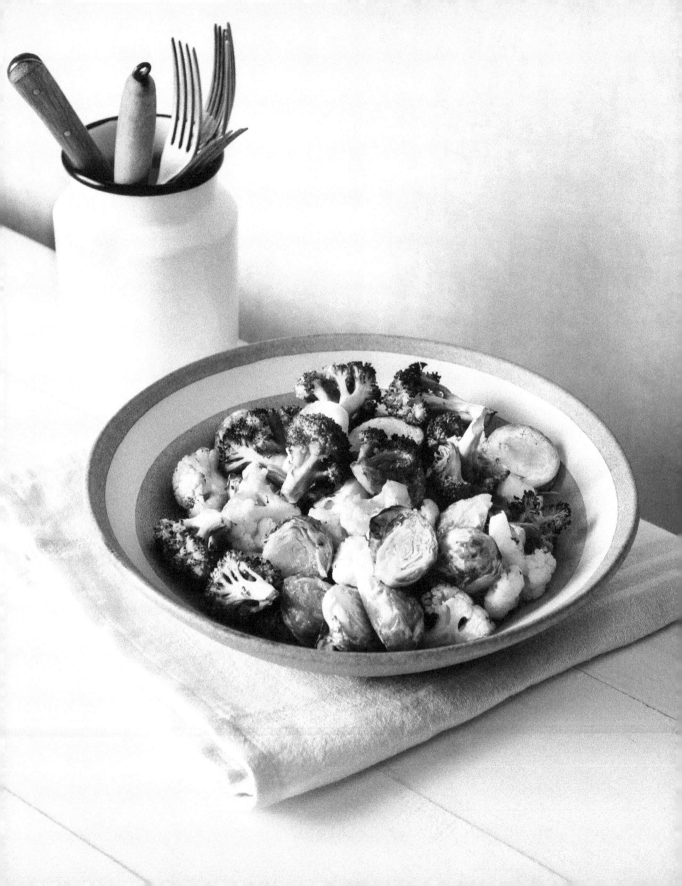

Sides

....
Roasted Veggies, page 125

Cauliflower "Rice"

Rice is a staple food all over the world, both as a side dish and as the main source of carbohydrates. The keto lifestyle does not recommend eating rice, so cauliflower "rice" takes its place in many households following it. Chopped, cooked cauliflower has an almost identical texture to cooked basmati rice. You must watch the cooking time carefully because overcooking the cauliflower will leave you with a mushy mess. If you overcook the cauliflower, mash it up instead with cream and a dollop of butter for mashed "potatoes."

Serves 4 | **Prep time: 15 minutes** | **Cook time: 5 minutes**

VEGETARIAN, NUT FREE, DAIRY FREE, GLUTEN FREE, PALEO

5 cups chopped cauliflower

2 teaspoons extra-virgin olive oil

1 teaspoon minced garlic

2 tablespoons water

1. In a food processor, pulse the cauliflower until finely chopped.

2. In a large skillet over medium heat, heat the olive oil. Sauté the garlic until fragrant and softened, about 2 minutes.

3. Add the cauliflower and water to the skillet. Cover the skillet, and steam the cauliflower until tender crisp, about 2 minutes.

4. Transfer the cauliflower to a bowl; serve hot.

VARIATION *This quick, mild-tasting dish has a similar texture to real rice, and the mild flavor lends itself well to interesting recipe additions. You can add vegetables, chopped meats, spices, soy sauce, salsa, chopped nuts, fresh herbs, or hot spices to the basic cauliflower "rice" dish, depending on your palate and culinary needs.*

Per Serving Calories: 65; Total Fat: 5g, 70%; Protein: 3g, 6%; Total Carbs: 5g; Fiber: 3g; Net Carbs: 3g, 24%; Sugar: 3g

Baked Parmesan Tomatoes

Think of this as a baked version of a caprese salad—tomatoes, Parmesan, and basil served up in a warm, melty way that you will love.

Serves 2 | **Prep time: 5 minutes** | **Cook time: 10 minutes**

VEGETARIAN, NUT FREE, GLUTEN FREE

1 large tomato, cut into 4 slices

1 teaspoon Italian seasoning

½ cup shaved Parmesan

1 teaspoon sliced fresh basil

1. Preheat the oven to 400°F. Line a baking sheet with parchment paper or a silicone baking mat.

2. On the prepared baking sheet, arrange the tomatoes in a single layer. Sprinkle with the Italian seasoning and top with the Parmesan and basil.

3. Bake until the cheese is bubbling, about 10 minutes.

. . . .

Per Serving Calories: 124; Total Fat: 7g, 52%; Protein: 10g, 35%; Total Carbs: 5g; Fiber: 1g; Net Carbs: 4g, 13%

Sautéed Spinach with Garlic

Here is garlicky and delicious side that goes hand-in-hand with essentially any main dish. Not only is this recipe quick and easy (about 10 minutes altogether), but it's also packed with flavor. And if you want even more flavor, try the variations by adding either cheese or bacon.

Serves 4 | **Prep time: 5 minutes** | **Cook time: 10 minutes**

VEGETARIAN, NUT FREE, GLUTEN FREE, PALEO

2 tablespoons unsalted butter or extra-virgin olive oil

¼ white onion, diced

3 garlic cloves, sliced

12 ounces fresh spinach

Salt

Freshly ground black pepper

1. In a large skillet over medium heat, melt the butter.

2. Add the onion and garlic. Cook for 5 to 7 minutes until the onion is softened and translucent.

3. Add the spinach and reduce the heat to medium low. Season well with salt and pepper. Cook for 3 to 4 minutes or until the spinach wilts. Serve immediately.

CHEESE VARIATION *Add ¼ cup grated Parmesan to the spinach before serving. Stir well to combine.*

BACON VARIATION *Cook 2 or 3 bacon slices in the skillet before adding the garlic and onion. Remove the bacon and crumble it. Add the spinach and return the bacon to the skillet. Stir well to combine.*

....

Per Serving Calories: 75; Total Fat: 6g, 71%; Protein: 3g, 9%; Total Carbs: 4g; Fiber: 2g; Net Carbs: 2g, 20%; Sugar: 1g

Cheese Variation Per Serving Calories: 102; Total Fat: 8g, 67%; Protein: 5g, 17%; Total Carbs: 5g; Fiber: 2g; Net Carbs: 3g, 16%; Sugar: 1g

Bacon Variation Per Serving Calories: 171; Total Fat: 16g, 81%; Protein: 5g, 10%; Total Carbs: 4g; Fiber: 2g; Net Carbs: 2g, 9%; Sugar: 1g

Parmesan & Pork Rind Green Beans

Consider this a keto update on the traditional green bean casserole. Drizzled in olive oil and seasoned with a bit of salt plus the Parmesan cheese and pork rinds, the roasted beans are bursting with flavor.

Serves 2 | **Prep time: 5 minutes** | **Cook time: 15 minutes**

NUT FREE, GLUTEN FREE

½ pound fresh green beans

2 tablespoons crushed pork rinds

2 tablespoons olive oil

1 tablespoon grated Parmesan cheese

Pink Himalayan salt

Freshly ground black pepper

1. Preheat the oven to 400°F.

2. In a medium bowl, combine the green beans, pork rinds, olive oil, and Parmesan cheese. Season with pink Himalayan salt and pepper, and toss until the beans are thoroughly coated.

3. Spread the bean mixture on a baking sheet in a single layer, and roast for about 15 minutes. At the halfway point, give the pan a little shake to move the beans around, or just give them a stir.

4. Divide the beans between two plates and serve.

INGREDIENT TIP *You can use any flavor of pork rinds to add additional zest to the green beans.*

Per Serving Calories: 175; Total Fat: 15g, 74%; Saturated Fat: 4g; Protein: 6g, 12%; Total Carbs: 8g, 14%; Fiber: 3g; Net Carbs: 5g; Cholesterol: 34mg

Sautéed Cabbage

Cabbage is often overlooked and gets pushed to the back of the fridge, but once you learn how versatile (and cheap!) it is, you'll find yourself adding it to your meal plans almost every week. This simple preparation can complement any meal.

Serves 4 | **Prep time: 5 minutes** | **Cook time: 15 minutes**

VEGETARIAN, NUT FREE, DAIRY FREE, GLUTEN FREE, PALEO, ONE POT

¼ cup (½ stick) salted
   butter or ghee
1 head cabbage, chopped
3 tablespoons apple
   cider vinegar
Salt
Freshly ground black pepper

1. In a large pot over medium heat, melt the butter. Add the shredded cabbage and cook, stirring occasionally, until the cabbage is tender. If you like it with a little crunch, cook it for 10 to 12 minutes. If you want yours more tender, cook it a few minutes longer.

2. Add the vinegar, season with salt and pepper, and serve hot.

VARIATION *You can really change the flavor of this simple dish by adding different spices, such as cumin, coriander, and/or crushed red pepper. Go ahead and experiment with other flavors that you like.*

....

Per Serving Calories: 158; Total Fat: 12g; Saturated Fat: 17g, 63%; Protein: 3g, 7%; Total Carbs: 12g; Fiber: 5g; Net Carbs: 7g, 30%; Cholesterol: 31mg

Roasted Cauliflower with Prosciutto, Capers & Almonds

This is perfect as a side with any meat, but it can also stand on its own as a light dinner or hearty lunch. The capers are probably the best part; they provide a nice pop of flavor, and the slivered almonds give it a surprising crunch. For extra protein, throw a couple of seasoned chicken breasts into the pan with the cauliflower.

Serves 2 | **Prep time: 5 minutes** | **Cook time: 25 minutes**

GLUTEN FREE, ONE PAN

12 ounces cauliflower florets (you can find pre-cut florets in the produce section of most grocery stores)

2 tablespoons leftover bacon grease or olive oil

Pink Himalayan salt

Freshly ground black pepper

2 ounces sliced prosciutto, torn into small pieces

¼ cup slivered almonds

2 tablespoons capers

2 tablespoons grated Parmesan cheese

1. Preheat the oven to 400°F. Line a baking pan with a silicone baking mat or parchment paper.

2. Put the cauliflower florets in the prepared baking pan with the bacon grease, and season with pink Himalayan salt and pepper. Or if you are using olive oil instead, drizzle the cauliflower with olive oil and season with pink Himalayan salt and pepper.

3. Roast the cauliflower for 15 minutes.

4. Stir the cauliflower so all sides are coated with the bacon grease.

5. Distribute the prosciutto pieces in the pan. Then add the slivered almonds and capers. Stir to combine. Sprinkle the Parmesan cheese on top, and roast for 10 minutes more.

6. Divide between two plates, using a slotted spoon so you don't get excess grease in the plates, and serve.

SUBSTITUTION TIP *Sliced green olives work well if you don't have capers.*

....

Per Serving Calories: 288; Total Fat: 24g, 75%; Saturated Fat: 5g; Protein: 14g, 17%; Total Carbs: 7g, 8%; Fiber: 3g; Net Carbs: 4g; Cholesterol: 20mg

Mushrooms with Camembert

Mushrooms have an interesting, almost meaty texture, and they tend to soak up all the flavorings in a recipe. Mushrooms are very high in vitamin D, the only vegetable source of this nutrient, and are an excellent source of potassium and selenium. Mushrooms can help reduce your cravings for sweet foods and help prevent spikes in blood sugar that can cause overeating.

Serves 4 | **Prep time: 5 minutes** | **Cook time: 15 minutes**

VEGETARIAN, NUT FREE, GLUTEN FREE, ONE PAN

2 tablespoons unsalted butter

2 teaspoons minced garlic

1 pound button
   mushrooms, halved

4 ounces Camembert
   cheese, diced

Freshly ground black pepper

1. Place a large skillet over medium-high heat and melt the butter. Add the garlic and sauté until translucent, about 3 minutes.

2. Add the mushrooms and sauté until they are tender, about 10 minutes.

3. Stir in the cheese and sauté until it is completely melted, about 2 minutes.

4. Season with pepper and serve hot.

. . . .

Per Serving Calories: 161; Total Fat: 13g, 70%; Protein: 9g, 21%; Total Carbs: 4g; Fiber: 1g; Net Carbs: 3g, 9%

Roasted Veggies

You can roast pretty much any vegetable! Cauliflower, broccoli, and Brussels sprouts are especially delicious when cooked this way, but feel free to experiment with your favorites. Just make sure you chop the vegetables into pieces that are about the same size so they roast evenly.

Makes 4 servings | **Prep time: 5 minutes** | **Cook time: 20 to 25 minutes**

VEGETARIAN, NUT FREE, DAIRY FREE, GLUTEN FREE, PALEO, ONE PAN

1 cup cauliflower florets

1 cup broccoli florets

1 cup Brussels sprouts

2 tablespoons extra-virgin olive oil

Salt

Freshly ground black pepper

1. Preheat the oven to 425°F.

2. In a medium bowl, toss the cauliflower, broccoli, and Brussels sprouts with olive oil, and season with salt and pepper.

3. On a baking sheet, spread the vegetables in a single layer. Be careful not to crowd them or the vegetables might steam rather than roast.

4. Cook the vegetables for 20 to 25 minutes, stirring once about halfway through.

5. Sprinkle with a little more salt and pepper before serving.

VARIATION *Another great mix of vegetables is green beans, zucchini, asparagus, and bell peppers. This mix needs to roast for only about 15 minutes—otherwise, prepare it the same way.*

Per Serving Calories: 83; Total Fat: 7g, 74%; Protein: 2g, 6%; Total Carbs: 5g; Fiber: 2g; Net Carbs: 3g, 20%

Sautéed Crispy Zucchini

Anyone who has eaten a grilled cheese sandwich or picked the crispy edges off of a lasagna knows how incredible these cheesy bits taste. That rich golden crisp cheese is what you end up with on your sautéed zucchini when you prepare this recipe. The trick is to let the ingredients sit in the skillet after you add the cheese so it has the chance to melt and lightly caramelize before stirring.

Serves 4 | **Prep time: 15 minutes** | **Cook time: 10 minutes**

VEGETARIAN, NUT FREE, GLUTEN FREE, ONE PAN

2 tablespoons unsalted butter

4 zucchini, cut into
   ¼-inch-thick rounds

½ cup freshly grated
   Parmesan cheese

Freshly ground black pepper

1. Place a large skillet over medium-high heat and melt the butter.

2. Add the zucchini and sauté until tender and lightly browned, about 5 minutes.

3. Spread the zucchini evenly in the skillet and sprinkle the Parmesan cheese over the vegetables.

4. Cook without stirring until the Parmesan cheese is melted and crispy where it touches the skillet, about 5 minutes. Serve hot.

. . . .

Per Serving Calories: 94; Total Fat: 8g, 76%; Protein: 4g, 20%; Total Carbs: 1g; Fiber: 0g; Net Carbs: 1g, 4%

Thai Peanut Roasted Cauliflower

Peanut butter is a controversial keto food, since peanuts are a legume, but if you use a no-sugar-added brand or make your own Homemade Nut Butter (see page 28), you can certainly enjoy it in moderation. This is another side dish that stand on its own as a light lunch or dinner.

Serves 2 | **Prep time: 10 minutes** | **Cook time: 20 minutes**

VEGETARIAN, DAIRY FREE, GLUTEN FREE

½ head cauliflower, cut into bite-size florets

1 tablespoon extra-virgin olive oil

Salt

Freshly ground black pepper

½ cup unsweetened full-fat coconut milk

2 tablespoons peanut butter

¼ teaspoon red curry paste

1 garlic clove, minced

1 tablespoon chopped fresh parsley or dried

1. Preheat the oven to 400°F.

2. On a baking sheet, arrange the cauliflower in a single layer. Drizzle with the olive oil and season with salt and pepper. Roast for about 20 minutes, until the edges are brown.

3. While the cauliflower is cooking, in a blender, combine the coconut milk, peanut butter, curry paste, and garlic. Process until smooth.

4. Once the cauliflower is finished, divide it between two plates and drizzle the peanut sauce on top. Garnish with the parsley.

SUBSTITUTION TIP *Switch it up by using your own Homemade Nut Butter (page 28).*

Per Serving Calories: 290; Total Fat: 27g, 80%; Protein: 8g, 9%; Total Carbs: 9g, 11%; Fiber: 3g; Net Carbs: 6g

Sautéed Asparagus with Walnuts

If you are a foodie, you probably wait with anticipation for spring and the slender, elegant asparagus spears that come into season at that time. Asparagus is a good choice for keto followers because although this veggie contains carbs, it is also very high in fiber, which creates a low net carb result. Asparagus is an antioxidant and anti-inflammatory, so it is excellent for eye health, helps fight cancers, and is wonderful for your heart.

Serves 4 | **Prep time: 10 minutes** | **Cook time: 5 minutes**

VEGETARIAN, DAIRY FREE, GLUTEN FREE, ONE PAN

1½ tablespoons olive oil

¾ pound asparagus, woody ends trimmed

Sea salt

Freshly ground pepper

¼ cup chopped walnuts

1. Place a large skillet over medium-high heat and add the olive oil.

2. Sauté the asparagus until the spears are tender and lightly browned, about 5 minutes. Season with salt and pepper.

3. Remove the skillet from the heat, and toss the asparagus with the walnuts. Serve hot.

. . . .

Per Serving Calories: 124; Total Fat: 12g, 81%; Protein: 3g, 9%; Total Carbs: 4g; Fiber: 2g; Net Carbs: 2g, 10%

Roasted Radishes with Brown Butter Sauce

These warm, buttery roasted radishes look and taste like baby red potatoes. They are crispy on the outside, warm and smooth on the inside. The brown butter sauce makes this dish truly delicious.

Serves 2 | **Prep time: 10 minutes** | **Cook time: 15 minutes**

VEGETARIAN, NUT FREE, GLUTEN FREE, PALEO

2 cups halved radishes

1 tablespoon olive oil

Pink Himalayan salt

Freshly ground black pepper

2 tablespoons unsalted butter

1 tablespoon chopped fresh flat-leaf Italian parsley

1. Preheat the oven to 450°F.

2. In a medium bowl, toss the radishes in the olive oil and season with pink Himalayan salt and pepper.

3. Spread the radishes on a baking sheet in a single layer. Roast for 15 minutes, stirring halfway through.

4. Meanwhile, when the radishes have been roasting for about 10 minutes, in a small, light-colored saucepan over medium heat, melt the butter completely, stirring frequently, and season with pink Himalayan salt. When the butter begins to bubble and foam, continue stirring. When the bubbling diminishes a bit, the butter should be a nice nutty brown. The browning process should take about 3 minutes total. Transfer the browned butter to a heat-safe container (such as a mug).

5. Remove the radishes from the oven, and divide them between two plates. Spoon the brown butter over the radishes, top with the chopped parsley, and serve.

INGREDIENT TIP *You can keep the stems on the radishes to roast them if you prefer them that way.*

Per Serving Calories: 181; Total Fat: 19g, 93%; Saturated Fat: 8g; Protein: 1g, 2%; Total Carbs: 4g, 5%; Fiber: 2g; Net Carbs: 2g; Cholesterol: 31mg

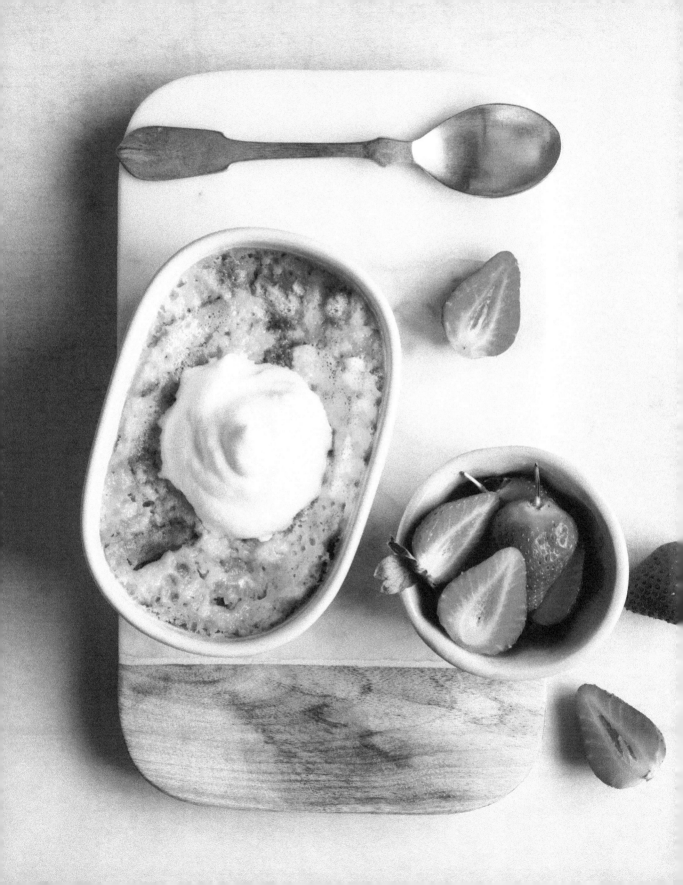

Drinks & Dessert

Strawberries & Cream Cake, page 142

Root Beer Float

Cutting sugar and carbs from your diet doesn't mean you have to miss out on old-school treats like root beer floats. This version is keto-friendly, and you won't miss the sugar at all.

Serves 2 | **Prep time: 5 minutes**

VEGETARIAN, NUT FREE, GLUTEN FREE, ONE BOWL

1 (12-ounce) can diet root beer (such as Zevia's)

4 tablespoons heavy (whipping) cream

1 teaspoon vanilla extract

6 ice cubes

1. In a food processor (or blender), combine the root beer, cream, vanilla, and ice.

2. Blend well, pour into two tall glasses, and serve with a bendy straw.

VARIATION *If you are looking for a boozy root beer float, you can add vanilla vodka or rum to this mix.*

. . . .

Per Serving Calories: 56; Total Fat: 6g, 92%; Saturated Fat: 7g; Protein: 1g, 2%; Total Carbs: 3g, 6%; Fiber: 0g; Net Carbs: 3g; Cholesterol: 41mg

Chocolate Raspberry Cheesecake Shake

If cheesecake is your weakness, why not drink it, too? This shake includes all the luxurious ingredients of a cheesecake, whipped up into a frothy, straw-worthy drink.

Serves 1 | Prep time: 5 minutes

VEGETARIAN, NUT FREE, ONE BOWL

1 cup unsweetened almond milk

1 tablespoon organic heavy (whipping) cream

1 tablespoon organic cream cheese, at room temperature

⅓ cup low-carb vanilla or graham cracker whey protein powder

½ cup raspberries

2 ice cubes

In a blender, combine the almond milk, heavy cream, cream cheese, protein powder, raspberries, and ice cubes. Blend until smooth, and pour into a tall glass to serve.

....

Per Serving Calories: 251; Total Fat: 15g; Saturated Fat: 6g, 54%; Protein: 25g, 40%; Total Carbs: 9g; Fiber: 5g; Net Carbs: 4g, 6%; Cholesterol: 87mg

Keto-Jito

When dessert time really means cocktail time, here is a keto-friendly take on the mojito. Of course, cocktails don't have any nutritional value, but it's still good to have low-carb options when you're entertaining.

Serves 1 | Prep time: 5 minutes

VEGETARIAN, NUT FREE, DAIRY FREE, GLUTEN FREE, PALEO, ONE BOWL

¼ cup loosely packed fresh mint leaves

1 ounce freshly squeezed lime juice

1 teaspoon confectioners' erythritol

1 cup ice

2 ounces white rum

4 ounces club soda

1. In a tall glass, muddle the mint using the handle of a wooden spoon.

2. Add the lime juice and erythritol, and mix.

3. Add the ice and then pour in the rum and club soda. Stir again.

VARIATION *I also like to muddle blackberries into this for an extra-special keto-jito.*

....

Per Serving Calories: 130; Total Fat: 0g, 0%; Protein: 0g, 0%; Total Carbs: 1g; Fiber: 0g; Net Carbs: 1g; 100%

Raspberry Cheesecake Fluff

Craving something sweet? This decadent Raspberry Cheesecake Fluff will do the trick and leave you guilt-free! You can also use this fluff to top any warm mug cake, keto-approved cheesecake, or a fresh bowl of berries.

Serves 4 | Prep time: 5 minutes

VEGETARIAN, NUT FREE, ONE BOWL

1 cup heavy (whipping) cream

8 ounces cream cheese, at room temperature

4 ounces raspberries

½ cup sugar substitute (such as Swerve)

1 teaspoon vanilla extract

Pinch salt

1. In blender or in a bowl using a hand mixer, whip the cream to stiff peaks, 2 to 4 minutes.

2. Add the cream cheese, raspberries, sugar substitute, vanilla, and salt, and blend until smooth and well combined.

. . . .

Per Serving Calories: 417; Total Fat: 41g; Saturated Fat: 25g, 88%; Protein: 5g, 5%; Total Carbs: 7g; Fiber: 2g; Net Carbs: 5g, 7%; Cholesterol: 143mg

Keto "Rice" Pudding

This is a great choice for when you're looking for volume and want to feel that "fullness" without extra calories and carbs. Shirataki "rice" is made from the konjac plant, traditionally used in Japanese cuisine and Chinese medicine. The "rice" is 97 percent water and 3 percent soluble fiber. It's filling due to the high water and fiber content and absorbs the flavors of any dish you pair it with. When you first open the package, you'll notice it has an off-putting smell, but don't worry, the smell goes away once you drain and rinse it.

Serves 2 | **Prep time: 5 minutes** | **Cook time: 7 minutes**

VEGETARIAN, NUT FREE, DAIRY FREE, GLUTEN FREE, PALEO, ONE PAN

1 (8-ounce) bag shirataki "rice," thoroughly rinsed and drained

1 scoop flavored MCT powder or collagen powder

Pinch Himalayan sea salt

Pinch ground cinnamon

TOPPING SUGGESTIONS

1 tablespoon sugar-free whipped cream

1 tablespoon chopped nuts (pili nuts, macadamia nuts, walnuts, pecans, almonds)

1 tablespoon chopped dark chocolate or stevia-sweetened chocolate chips

1 tablespoon sugar-free maple syrup

1. In a small saucepan, bring 1 cup of water to a boil. When the water begins to boil, add the shirataki "rice" and cook for 2 minutes. Drain in a colander and return to the saucepan.

2. Let any remaining water evaporate and then reduce the heat to medium. Add the MCT powder, salt, and cinnamon. Stir well and cook for another 3 to 5 minutes.

3. Pour into a bowl and add your desired toppings.

TIME-SAVING TIP *Double or triple the recipe and divide into small, airtight containers and store in the refrigerator for the week. When ready to eat, microwave for 30 to 60 seconds, add toppings, and enjoy.*

. . . .

Per Serving (½ recipe without toppings) Calories: 58; Total Fat: 4g, 62%; Saturated Fat: 1g; Protein: 1g, 8%; Total Carbs: 4.5g; Fiber: 4.5g; Net Carbs: 0g; Cholesterol: 6mg

5-Minute Chocolate Mousse

You'd never guess that this fluffy, whipped dessert is sugar-free or dairy-free! Full-fat coconut cream is a healthy, dairy-free alternative to heavy whipping cream. It adds delicious flavor to shakes, curries, soups, and ice cream, and here, it makes for a rich and chocolatey mousse.

Serves 4 | Prep time: 5 minutes

VEGETARIAN, NUT FREE, DAIRY FREE, GLUTEN FREE, PALEO, ONE BOWL

1 (14-ounce) can coconut cream, chilled

3 tablespoons unsweetened cocoa powder

¼ cup sugar substitute (such as Swerve)

1 teaspoon vanilla extract

1. In a large mixing bowl, whip the coconut cream with a hand mixer until fluffy, about 3 minutes. If you don't have a hand mixer, you can whip it in the blender.

2. Fold in the cocoa powder, sugar substitute, and vanilla and serve immediately.

VARIATION *Add half a ripe avocado to make the mousse even creamier!*

....

Per Serving Calories: 222; Total Fat: 22g; Saturated Fat: 21g, 89%; Protein: 1g, 2%; Total Carbs: 5g; Fiber: 1g; Net Carbs: 4g, 9%; Cholesterol: 0mg

Spiced Chocolate Fat Bombs

Good-quality cocoa powder is an acceptable ingredient on the keto diet, which means you can still enjoy a chocolate dessert and snack when you need a fix. Dark chocolate like cocoa is very high in manganese, magnesium, copper, iron, and fiber as well as antioxidants, which fight free radicals in the body. Dark chocolate has been found to help lower blood pressure, reduce cholesterol, and improve cognitive function.

Serves 12 │ **Prep time: 10 minutes** │ **Cook time: 4 minutes** │ **Chill time: 15 minutes**

VEGETARIAN, DAIRY FREE, GLUTEN FREE

¾ cup coconut oil

¼ cup cocoa powder

¼ cup almond butter

⅛ teaspoon chili powder

3 drops liquid stevia

1. Line a mini muffin tin with paper liners and set aside.

2. Put a small saucepan over low heat and add the coconut oil, cocoa powder, almond butter, chili powder, and stevia.

3. Heat until the coconut oil is melted, then whisk to blend.

4. Spoon the mixture into the muffin cups and place the tin in the refrigerator until the bombs are firm, about 15 minutes.

5. Transfer the cups to an airtight container and store the fat bombs in the freezer until you want to serve them.

. . . .

Per Serving (1 fat bomb) Calories: 117; Total Fat: 12g, 92%; Protein: 2g, 4%; Total Carbs: 2g; Fiber: 0g; Net Carbs: 2g, 4%

Coconut Truffles

Unsweetened coconut flakes wrap around rich cream cheese for these quick and easy truffles. Extremely simple, these can be frozen and thawed as needed or refrigerated in an airtight container. Experiment by adding spices, like cinnamon, for a twist.

Serves 12 | **Prep time: 25 minutes**

VEGETARIAN, NUT FREE, GLUTEN FREE

8 ounces (1 package) cream cheese, at room temperature

½ cup stevia, or other sugar substitute

2 teaspoons coconut extract

½ cup unsweetened shredded coconut

1. In a medium bowl, mix together the cream cheese, stevia, and coconut extract.

2. Scoop into balls, 1 to 2 tablespoons in size. It should yield about 12.

3. Roll the balls in the coconut flakes. Chill the truffles for 15 minutes before serving.

....

Per Serving (1 truffle) Calories: 98; Total Fat: 9.3g, 82%; Saturated Fat: 5g; Protein: 1.8g, 10%; Total Carbs: 1.6g, 8%; Fiber: 0.7g; Net Carbs: 0.9g; Cholesterol: 21mg

Chewy Chocolate Chip Cookies

If you love puffy, chewy chocolate chip cookies, these will be your go-to keto replacement, studded with sugar-free, keto-friendly chocolate chips. Nuts are also a great addition, too, if you like.

Serves 10 | **Prep time: 10 minutes** | **Cook time: 5 minutes**

VEGETARIAN, GLUTEN FREE

¼ cup unsalted butter

1¼ cups almond flour

¼ teaspoon salt

¼ cup erythritol

¼ teaspoon cream of tartar

1 large egg

1 teaspoon vanilla extract

¼ cup sugar-free chocolate chips

1. Preheat the oven to 350°F.

2. Line a baking sheet with parchment paper or a silicone baking mat and set aside.

3. In a saucepan or in the microwave, melt the butter. Place in a room-temperature container and let it set in the refrigerator for 10 minutes to cool down.

4. In a large bowl, combine the almond flour, salt, erythritol, and cream of tartar. Stir to combine.

5. In a small bowl, combine the egg, vanilla, and cooled butter. Whisk together.

6. Pour the wet ingredients into the dry ingredients and combine everything together with a large spoon or rubber scraper, then fold in the chocolate chips.

7. Scoop 2- to 3-inch mounds of cookie dough onto the prepared baking sheet, and use your hands or the back of the spoon to flatten them a bit.

8. Bake the cookies for 10 to 12 minutes, until the edges turn golden brown.

9. Let the cookies cool for 10 to 15 minutes before transferring them to a cooling rack to cool for an additional 15 minutes before serving.

Per Serving Calories: 121; Total Fat: 9g, 83%; Protein: 2g, 7%; Total Carbs: 3g; Fiber: 1g; Net Carbs: 2g, 10%

Peanut Butter Cookies

Peanut butter and cream cheese come together to create this unique, chewy cookie. Crunchy on the outside but chewy on the inside, these mimic the traditional peanut butter cookie in many ways. The dough will be very sticky, so wet your hands before forming the cookies.

Serves 25 | **Prep time: 10 minutes** | **Cook time: 13 minutes**

VEGETARIAN, GLUTEN FREE

1 cup sugar-free peanut butter

½ cup cream cheese, at room temperature

20 drops liquid stevia, or other liquid sugar substitute

1 egg

1 teaspoon pure vanilla extract

1. Preheat the oven to 350°F.

2. In a large bowl, combine the peanut butter, cream cheese, stevia, egg, and vanilla. Mix thoroughly to combine. Divide the dough by heaping tablespoons into 25 equal portions. Form into balls.

3. On parchment-lined baking sheets, arrange the cookie balls at least 1 inch apart.

4. With a fork, flatten each cookie, crisscrossing the imprint with the tines.

5. Place the baking sheets in the oven. Bake for 12 to 13 minutes, or until golden brown.

6. Cool the cookies for 2 to 3 minutes before serving. Store in an airtight container.

. . . .

Per Serving (1 cookie) Calories: 79; Total Fat: 6.9g, 79%; Saturated Fat: 2g; Protein: 3.1g, 13%; Total Carbs: 2.2g, 8%; Fiber: 0.6g; Net Carbs: 1.6g; Cholesterol: 12mg

Strawberries & Cream Cake

Make this sweet, creamy cake in the spring when plump strawberries arrive at the market. It makes for the perfect dessert, of course, but you can also enjoy it for breakfast when you want something indulgent to start the day.

Serves 1 | **Prep time: 10 minutes** | **Cook time: 4 minutes**

VEGETARIAN, GLUTEN FREE

2 large free-range eggs

¼ cup low- to zero-carb vanilla syrup (see Ingredient Tip)

2 tablespoons Golden Ghee (page 27), melted but not hot

2 tablespoons organic cream cheese, at room temperature

¼ cup almond flour

4 strawberries, hulled and cut into chunks

¼ cup sugar-free whipped cream

1. In a single-serving blender, blend the eggs, vanilla syrup, ghee, and cream cheese until well mixed. Scrape the mixture into a small microwave-safe bowl or mug.

2. Stir in the almond flour, then stir in the strawberries.

3. Microwave the batter on high for 4 minutes. Let the cake cool for a minute, then top it with the whipped cream.

INGREDIENT TIP *The vanilla sweetener makes all the difference in this recipe. You can find it online and at specialty grocery stores. Look for the brands Torani (made with Splenda) and Monin (made with Splenda and erythritol).*

. . . .

Per Serving Calories: 719; Total Fat: 67g; Saturated Fat: 31g, 84%; Protein: 15g, 11%; Total Carbs: 10g; Fiber: 4g; Net Carbs: 6g, 5%; Cholesterol: 456mg;

Blueberry-Lemon Cake

In this cake, blueberry and lemon converge to create a bright, sweet flavor, and cream cheese helps create the perfect texture. A few blueberries go a long way, so don't overdo it or the bottom of your cake will be mushy.

Serves 8 | **Prep time: 10 minutes** | **Cook time: 20 minutes**

VEGETARIAN, NUT FREE, GLUTEN FREE

Nonstick cooking spray

2 tablespoons butter, cut into 4 pieces, plus more if desired

4 large eggs

4 ounces cream cheese

¼ cup coconut flour

¼ cup erythritol

1½ teaspoons baking powder

1 teaspoon vanilla extract

1 tablespoon lemon zest

¼ cup blueberries, fresh or frozen

1. Preheat the oven to 425°F. Coat an 8-by-8-inch baking pan with cooking spray.

2. Put the 4 pieces of butter in the baking pan and place the pan in the oven for 2 to 3 minutes to melt the butter, but make sure it doesn't brown or burn. Remove from the oven.

3. In a food processor, mixer, or blender, process the eggs, cream cheese, coconut flour, erythritol, baking powder, vanilla, and lemon zest until thoroughly combined.

4. Pour the batter into the baking pan with the melted butter.

5. Drop the blueberries into the cake, evenly spreading them throughout.

6. Bake for 15 minutes, or until a toothpick inserted into the center comes out clean.

7. Serve warm and add more butter on top, if you wish.

....

Per Serving Calories: 147; Total Fat: 11g, 72%; Protein: 5g, 14%; Total Carbs: 5g; Fiber: 3g; Net Carbs: 2g, 14%; Erythritol: 2g

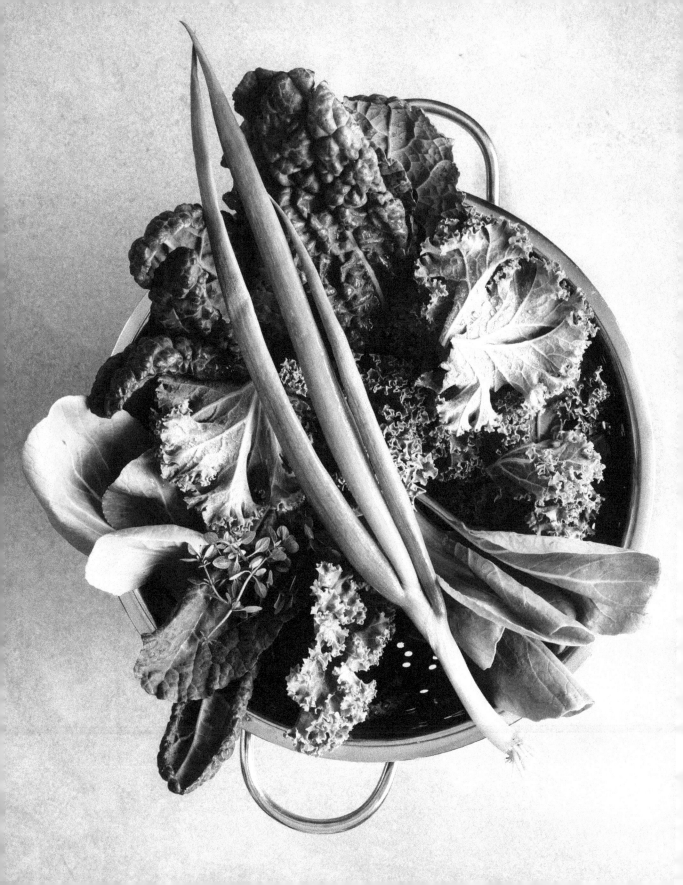

ADVICE FOR GOING OUT TO EAT

Getting rid of all culinary temptations is great for eating at home, but what happens when you go out to eat? Staying on a low-carb diet might seem difficult at first, but it can be easy with these few tips and a little bit of practice!

BREAKFAST

Skip the bagels, pancakes, Belgian waffles, French toast, or anything of the like. Opt for an omelet, or a few eggs with a side of sausage or ham. Skip the toast and hash browns.

LUNCH

Get a salad with lots of meat. Try a Cobb, chicken Caesar, or garden salad with chicken on top. Use plenty of olive oil and salt (electrolytes). You'll feel great afterward and have plenty of energy to last you until dinner. Carbs are why people get sleepy after lunch. Don't be a victim!

DINNER

When ordering a burger, ask to have it wrapped in lettuce. If they're unable to do that, just ask for no bun. If they bring the bun, take the patty and anything else off the bun and put it to the side. Skip the ketchup as well—it's full of sugar. Try mayo, mustard, red pepper sauce, sriracha, or any other low-carb sauce.

At Italian restaurants, skip the pasta and pizza, and order the protein-based dinners. Make sure to request salad or any other low-carb alternatives instead of the usual high-carb sides. If all else fails, just eat the topping off of the pizza and avoid the crust.

With Mexican cuisine, try to get your food in a bowl instead of in a burrito wrap or tortilla. Don't get rice or beans; instead, get extra sour cream and guacamole.

SIDES

French fries, steak fries, mashed potatoes, baked potatoes, rice, beans, corn on the cob, banana bread, and any other high-carb sides can be replaced with salad, asparagus, broccoli, green beans, or other low-carb vegetables. Most restaurants have some sort of salad for you to choose from. Make sure to always ask and double-check with the waiter or staff.

Instead of juice or soda, stick to water, tea, and coffee. Use heavy cream or half-and-half instead of milk.

In addition to fat, carbs, and protein, alcohol is also a macronutrient. It provides 7 calories per gram, the second most after fat, which provides 9 calories per gram. It is burned by the body before all the other macronutrients. If you drink too much alcohol, you will slow down your fat-burning process and impede your weight loss, if that is your goal.

If you're ordering alcohol, stay away from any cocktails, as they're all loaded with sugar. Dry or semidry wine has about 3 grams of carbs per glass, and low-carb beers like Michelob Ultra and Modelo have 3 to 4 grams of carbs per bottle. All pure spirits like vodka, Cognac, brandy, bourbon, whisky, rum, tequila, and gin are zero carbs. As always, drink in moderation, stay safe, and enjoy!

THE DIRTY DOZEN
& THE CLEAN FIFTEEN™

The Environmental Working Group (EWG) is a nonprofit, nonpartisan organization dedicated to protecting human health and the environment. Its mission is to empower people to live healthier lives in a healthier environment. This organization publishes an annual list of the twelve kinds of produce, in sequence, that have the highest amount of pesticide residue—the Dirty Dozen—as well as a list of the fifteen kinds of produce that have the least amount of pesticide residue—the Clean Fifteen. Please note that some of the foods listed here are not ideal for the keto diet (such as corn), but I'm presenting the EWG's list in its entirety.

THE DIRTY DOZEN

The 2018 Dirty Dozen* includes the following produce. These are considered among the year's most important produce to buy organic:

- Strawberries
- Apples
- Nectarines
- Peaches
- Celery
- Grapes
- Cherries
- Spinach
- Tomatoes
- Bell peppers
- Pears
- Potatoes

*The Dirty Dozen list contains two additional items—kale/collard greens and hot peppers—because they tend to contain trace levels of highly hazardous pesticides.

THE CLEAN FIFTEEN

The least critical to buy organically are the Clean Fifteen. The following are on the 2018 list:

- Avocados
- Corn**
- Pineapples
- Cabbage
- Sweet peas
- Onions
- Asparagus
- Mangos
- Papayas
- Kiwi
- Eggplant
- Honeydew
- Grapefruit
- Cantaloupe
- Cauliflower

** Some of the sweet corn sold in the United States is made from genetically engineered (GE) seed stock. Buy organic varieties of these crops to avoid GE produce.

KETO GLOSSARY

Understanding these terms clearly will contribute to your success with the ketogenic diet:

amino acids are the building blocks of the proteins the body needs to do everything from build muscle to grow hair and nails.

anabolic hormones stimulate protein synthesis, insulin production, and muscle growth.

BMR (basal metabolic rate) is the amount of energy expended while the body is at rest.

carbohydrates are organic compounds occurring in foods and living tissues and include sugars, starch, and cellulose. They can be broken down to release energy in the animal body.

cytokines are a broad and loose category of small proteins that are released by cells and affect the behavior of other cells.

electrolytes are minerals in your blood and other body fluids that affect the amount of water in your body, the acidity of your blood (pH), your muscle function, and other important processes.

glucose is a simple sugar that is considered to be an important energy source in living organisms and is a component of carbohydrates.

glycogen is a substance deposited in bodily tissues as a store of carbohydrates.

ketogenic or **keto** relates to the production of ketones in the body.

ketones are any of a class of organic compounds that burn fat when the body can't burn glucose for energy.

ketosis is the act of creating ketones while burning fat for energy.

lean mass weight or **lean body mass** is the amount your body weighs without fat.

macronutrients are substances such as fat or protein that your body requires in large amounts.

metabolism is the process by which your body converts the food and drink you consume into energy. During this complex biochemical process, calories in food and beverages are combined with oxygen to release the energy your body needs to function.

KETO DIET RESOURCES

WEBSITES AND BLOGS

Diet Doctor (dietdoctor.com) is a low-carb-focused site that provides articles and recipes as well as instructional videos and support.

Keto Diet App (ketodietapp.com) is a keto-only blog and a great resource for science-backed articles and recipes. It also has an app for mobile devices that includes recipes, articles, meal planning, and progress tracking.

Ketogenic.com is a comprehensive website that offers lots of detailed information about the science behind the ketogenic diet, plus recipes, podcasts, blog posts, forums, and its own macro calculator.

Keto In the City (ketointhecity.com) is where Jen Fisch shares keto recipes and tips on how to live a low-carb, high-fat life.

The Reddit Forum for Keto Dieters (reddit.com/r/keto) is a large community with hundreds of thousands of users who discuss progress, share cravings, and support each other.

Tasteaholics (tasteaholics.com) is a keto-centric website and resource that provides science-backed articles and recipes.

BOOKS

Coleman, Ella. *Keto Living Cookbook: Lose Weight with 101 Delicious and Low Carb Ketogenic Recipes.* New York, NY: Visual Magic Productions, 2013.

Davis, William, MD. *Wheat Belly: Lose the Wheat, Lose the Weight, and Find Your Path Back to Health.* New York, NY: Rodale Books, 2011.

Givens, Sara. *Ketogenic Diet Mistakes: You Wish You Knew.* Amazon Books, 2014.

McDonald, Lyle. *The Ketogenic Diet.* New York, NY: Morris Publishing, 1998.

Moore, Jimmy. *Keto Clarity: Your Definitive Guide to the Benefits of a Low-Carb, High-Fat Diet.* New York, NY: Victory Belt Publishing, 2014.

Taubes, Gary. *Good Calories, Bad Calories: Fats, Calories, and the Controversial Science of Diet and Health.* New York, NY: Anchor, 2008.

——. *Why We Get Fat: And What to Do About It.* New York, NY: Knopf, 2010.

Volek, Jeff S., and Stephen D. Phinney. *The Art and Science of Low Carbohydrate Performance.* New York, NY: Beyond Obesity LLC, 2012.

Keto Macro Calculators:

- **tasteaholics.com/keto-calculator** The simplest and most straightforward.
- **keto-calculator.ankerl.com** The most detailed and complex.
- **ketogains.com/ketogains-calculator** A simple calculator with no charts and only numbers.
- **MyFitnessPal (app)** A diet and exercise journal that provides meal tracking, calorie and macronutrient tracking, automatic calculation of meal nutrition, exercise tracking and caloric spend, and much more.

MEASUREMENTS & CONVERSIONS

Volume Equivalents (Liquid)

US Standard (ounces)	US Standard (approximate)	Metric
2 tablespoons	1 fluid ounce	30 milliliters
¼ cup	2 fluid ounces	60 milliliters
½ cup	4 fluid ounces	120 milliliters
1 cup	8 fluid ounces	240 milliliters
1½ cups	12 fluid ounces	355 milliliters
2 cups or 1 pint	16 fluid ounces	475 milliliters
4 cups or 1 quart	32 fluid ounces	1 liter
1 gallon	128 fluid ounces	4 liters

Oven Temperatures

Fahrenheit (F)	Celsius (C) (approximate)
250°F	120°C
300°F	150°C
325°F	165°C
350°F	180°C
375°F	190°C
400°F	200°C
425°F	220°C
450°F	230°C

Volume Equivalents (Dry)

US Standard	Metric (approximate)
⅛ teaspoon	½ milliliter
¼ teaspoon	1 milliliter
½ teaspoon	2 milliliters
¾ teaspoon	4 milliliters
1 teaspoon	5 milliliters
1 tablespoon	15 milliliters
¼ cup	59 milliliters
⅓ cup	79 milliliters
½ cup	118 milliliters
⅔ cup	156 milliliters
¾ cup	177 milliliters
1 cup	235 milliliters
2 cups or 1 pint	475 milliliters
3 cups	700 milliliters
4 cups or 1 quart	1 liter

Weight Equivalents

US Standard	Metric (approximate)
½ ounce	15 grams
1 ounce	30 grams
2 ounces	60 grams
4 ounces	115 grams
8 ounces	225 grams
12 ounces	340 grams
16 ounces or 1 pound	455 grams

RECIPE INDEX

INDEX

Ketogenic Diet

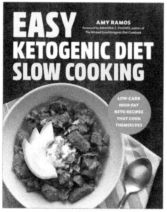

Easy Ketogenic Diet Slow Cooking

Low-Carb, High-Fat Keto Recipes that Cook Themselves

PAPERBACK 9781623159221 | EBOOK 9781623159238

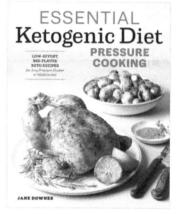

Essential Ketogenic Diet Pressure Cooking

Low-Effort, Big-Flavor Keto Recipes
for Any Pressure Cooker or Multicooker

PAPERBACK 9781939754400 | EBOOK 9781939754417

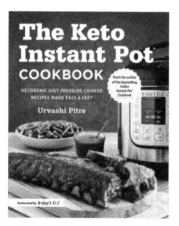

The Keto Instant Pot Cookbook

Ketogenic Diet Pressure Cooker Recipes Made Easy & Fast

PAPERBACK 9781641520430 | EBOOK 9781641520447

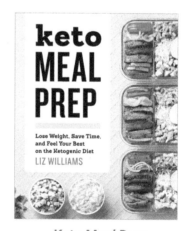

Keto Meal Prep

Lose Weight, Save Time, and Feel Your Best on the Ketogenic Diet

PAPERBACK 9781641522472 | EBOOK 9781641522489